CONTEMPORARY ISSUES in CRITICAL CARE NURSING VOLUME 4

Neonatal and Pediatric Critical Care Nursing

Edited by

Kit Stahler-Miller, M.S.N., R.N.
Instructor
Department of Nursing
LaSalle College
Philadelphia, Pennsylvania

Churchill Livingstone
NEW YORK, EDINBURGH, LONDON, AND MELBOURNE   1983

© Churchill Livingstone Inc. 1983

Distributed in the United Kingdom by Churchill Livingstone, Robert Stevenson House, 1-3 Baxter's Place, Leith Walk, Edinburgh EH1 3AF and by associated companies, branches and representatives throughout the world.

First published 1983

Printed in USA

ISBN 0-443-08174-3

7 6 5 4 3 2 1

Library of Congress Cataloging in Publication Data
Main entry under title:

Neonatal and pediatric critical care nursing.

   (Contemporary issues in critical care nursing ; 4)
   Bibliography: p.
   Includes index.
   1. Neonatal intensive care.   2. Pediatric intensive
care.   3. Intensive care nursing.   I. Stahler–Miller, Kit.
II. Series.   [DNLM: 1. Critical care—In infancy and
childhood.   2. Pediatric Nursing.   3. Infant, Newborn.
W1 C0769MQM v.4 / WY 159 N437]
RJ253.5.N45   1983   610.73'62   82-14676
ISBN 0-443-08174-3

This book is dedicated

To
The infants, children, families, nurses and others who
will benefit from this knowledge and sensitivity

To
Les Sampson, who provided me this opportunity

and

To
Neil, whose love and support sustained me
through this effort

Contributors

Philip A. Balderston, B.S.N., R.N., R.R.T.
Clinical Coordinator, Pediatric Intensive Care Unit, Department of
Respiratory Therapy, The Children's Hospital of Philadelphia, Philadelphia,
Pennsylvania; Formerly, Clinical Coordinator, Infant Intensive Care Unit,
The Children's Hospital of Philadelphia, Philadelphia, Pennsylvania

Lee B. Beerman, M.D., F.A.C.C.
Assistant Professor of Pediatrics, University of Pittsburgh School of
Medicine; Pediatric Cardiologist, Children's Hospital of Pittsburgh,
Pittsburgh, Pennsylvania

Mildred D. Boettcher, B.S.N., R.N.
Nursing Coordinator, Nutrition Support Service, The Children's Hospital of
Philadelphia, Philadelphia, Pennsylvania

Ruth A. Budd, M.S.N., R.N.C.
Transport Coordinator, Department of Nursing, Children's Hospital,
Columbus, Ohio; Formerly, Project Director, Comprehensive Care of the
Neonate, St. Christopher's Hospital for Children, Philadelphia, Pennsylvania

Elaine Dobbins, M.S.N., P.N.P., R.N.
Robert Wood Johnson Nurse Faculty Fellow, School of Nursing, University
of Maryland, Baltimore, Maryland

Mary E. Donar, B.S.N., R.N.
Head Nurse, Pediatric Intensive Care Unit—Intermediate, The Children's
Hospital of Philadelphia, Philadelphia, Pennsylvania

Julia M. Donlen, M.S.N., R.N.C.
Perinatal Nursing Instructor, Doctoral Candidate,
University of Pennsylvania, Philadelphia, Pennsylvania; Formerly, Neonatal
Nursing Instructor, Comprehensive Care of the Neonate Project, St.
Christopher's Hospital for Children, Philadelphia, Pennsylvania

Christine Garvey, B.S.N., R.N.
Assistant Head Nurse, Pediatric Critical Care Unit, Rush-Presbyterian—St.
Luke's Medical Center, Chicago, Illinois

Michael H. Gewitz, M.D.
Assistant Professor of Pediatrics, University of Pennsylvania School of
Medicine; Director, Pediatric Echocardiographic Laboratory, The Children's
Hospital of Philadelphia, Philadelphia, Pennsylvania

Marie Moore, R.N.
Assistant Head Nurse, Pediatric Critical Care Unit, Rush-Presbyterian—St.
Luke's Medical Center, Chicago, Illinois

Gilberto R. Pereira, M.D.
Assistant Professor of Pediatrics, University of Pennsylvania School of
Medicine; Staff Neonatologist, The Children's Hospital of Philadelphia,
Philadelphia, Pennsylvania

Eileen Pierce, M.S.N., R.N.
Unit Leader, Pediatric Critical Care Unit, Rush-Presbyterian—St. Luke's
Medical Center; Assistant Professor, College of Nursing, Rush University,
Chicago, Illinois

Barbara D. Schraeder, M.S.N., R.N.
Assistant Professor, Department of Baccalaureate Nursing, Thomas
Jefferson University; Doctoral Candidate, Temple University, Philadelphia,
Pennsylvania

Margaret C. Slota, M.N., R.N., C.C.R.N.
Instructor, Rutgers University College of Nursing; Clinical Nurse Specialist,
Children's Hospital of New Jersey, Newark, New Jersey; Formerly, Clinical
Nurse Specialist, Children's Hospital of Pittsburgh, Pittsburgh, Pennsylvania

Janet L. Snow, M.S.N., R.N.
Assistant Director of Administrative and Professional Practices, Chicago
Hospital Council; Doctoral Candidate, Rush University, Chicago, Illinois;
Formerly, Assistant Professor of Nursing, College of Nursing, Rush
University; Practitioner-Teacher, Pediatric Critical Care Unit, Rush-
Presbyterian—St. Luke's Medical Center, Chicago, Illinois

Alan R. Spitzer, M.D.
Assistant Professor of Pediatrics and Obstetrics and Gynecology, University
of Pennsylvania School of Medicine; Medical Director, Infant Transitional
Unit; Medical Director, Apnea Screening Program, The Children's Hospital
of Philadelphia, Philadelphia, Pennsylvania

Kit Stahler-Miller, M.S.N., R.N.
Instructor, Department of Nursing, LaSalle College, Philadelphia,
Pennsylvania; Formerly, Research Nurse, Division of Neonatology, The
Children's Hospital of Philadelphia, Philadelphia, Pennsylvania

Nancy Stanish, B.S.N., R.N.
Assistant Head Nurse, Pediatric Critical Care Unit, Rush-Presbyterian—St.
Luke's Medical Center, Chicago, Illinois

Foreword

Guest Editor, Kit Stahler-Miller, is a professional nurse who brings her expertise in clinical practice, writing, and research to this series. Ms. Stahler-Miller has consistently directed her professional commitment toward the nursing care of critically ill neonates and children. Now she is extending that commitment by helping other nurses and health professionals increase their knowledge and skill in these highly specialized areas of critical care. In this book, which is both timely and useful, Ms. Stahler-Miller has included data from her own work and that of other highly competent nurses and physicians.

Two current trends in the delivery of neonatal and pediatric health care make this book especially timely. The trends are: the increase in ambulatory care services and the regionalization of critical care. As the trend to increase ambulatory care services (including one-day surgery and early discharge programs) decreases the number of neonates and children hospitalized for minor problems, more bed space is becoming available for critically ill neonates and children. It is economically feasible and medically safe to regionalize this care. Thus the transport of critically ill neonates and children is increasing. As these trends continue, hospitals providing services to this critically ill, young population will have more beds filled with neonates and children who require the complex nursing care described here. In light of the current trends in the field, this book will be useful to nurses and other health professionals involved in planning and providing critical care and long term follow-up.

The critically ill neonate is the focus of the first half of the book. The emphasis on this very early age is appropriate because of the potential impact of neonatal problems on later development. The second half of the book is focused on the critically ill child. The ten chapters together provide very current, useful information on a diversity of very pertinent topics. Although the topics are diverse, the authors share the common view that critically ill neonates and children require highly skilled nursing care that is not only technologically safe, but also accounts for their physiological, psychological, sociocultural, and developmental needs.

Experienced nurses and nurses new to critical care will find the book useful in bridging the psychosocial gap that often exists in critical care units, while providing new technological and theoretical knowledge. This combination should encourage creative application of the material to the nursing care of critically ill neonates, children, and their families.

Susan Schaeffer Jay, R.N., Ph.D.

Preface

The care of critically ill neonates and children is a complex and unique challenge. This care spans a wide range of physiologic, psychologic, socio-cultural and developmental considerations, and includes the special aspect of caring for the family with a dependent member. The quality of this care is further dependent on the setting in which it is delivered, the availability and correct use of age-specific equipment and resources, and most importantly, the expertise and skill of the health care personnel involved in the care of the children. When all of these things are considered, excellence in the care of critically ill infants and children is dependent on a firm commitment to children and to their total care.

This book presents concepts and issues to stimulate thought, promote broad application, and catalyze change. The book contains an unusual variety of timely topics that are important to nurses involved in the management of critically ill infants and children. Although the book is not exhaustive, the carefully selected and diversely authored topics within each specialty are expansive, well-developed, and creative. Some chapters are issue-oriented, but most are strongly clinical and are therefore easily integrated into clinical practice. They emphasize current concepts of management, implications of therapy, and relevant research findings. Some chapters use theoretical frameworks to validate and strengthen the basis for nursing practice. Others include historical information and offer recommendations for change. Finally, the variety, expertise and combination of authors represent leadership and collaboration in health care delivery. All of these elements contribute interesting perspectives to this important and challenging field of critical care nursing.

This volume is written primarily for experienced neonatal and pediatric critical care nurses whose interests include consideration of issues related to research and clinical management, and to professional and societal health care trends. The content is also meaningful for graduate students in perinatal, pediatric, and critical care programs, and for undergraduate students in a pediatric elective. I hope that other readers will find this reference stimulating and applicable. Adult critical care nurses may notice the concepts that are applicable throughout the life cycle and appreciate some of the anatomic, physiologic, and psychologic aspects that are specific to infants and children. They may also appreciate the emphasis on providing holistic care and maintaining family and societal integrity. Nurses who are administrators, educators and researchers, and other interdisciplinary health care team members may find the viewpoints enlightening and challenging.

The book progresses from infancy to childhood and is divided into ten chapters. The book's tone is set by a presentation of a theoretical framework and nursing perspective of the low-birth-weight infant. This is followed by some of the primary problems, advances, and issues related to the high-risk neonate, including management of mechanical ventilation, patent ductus arteriosus and nutrition, and a view of trends and conflicts in perinatal research. The second half of the book focuses more on issues that affect the care of critically ill children, with the two specialties bridged by a thorough evaluation and analysis of the care and issues related to the child with chronic respiratory failure of infancy. The middle part of the book discusses improved survival of critically ill children after cardiac surgery and the nursing role in the perioperative period. This is followed by a chapter discussing transcultural nursing considerations related to the critically ill Vietnamese child and its family. The next chapter presents issues related to how and where critically ill children are cared for and the implications. The book concludes with a chapter describing successful implementation of primary nursing in a pediatric critical care unit.

Although these chapters can stand alone, they work well together; they build on and reinforce similar concepts and issues throughout the entirety—an exceptional quality from authors often unknown to each other and geographically widespread. This level of knowledge, conceptualization, reinforcement and practice says something very positive about the caliber of neonatal and pediatric critical care nursing.

The creation of this book has been a challenging and rewarding experience. My special thanks goes to the authors and to the anonymous reviewers for their interest, perseverance, and, in many cases, wise counsel.

Kit Stahler-Miller

Contents

Neonatal and Pediatric Critical Care Nursing

1 | The Low-birth-weight Infant: A Nursing Perspective

Julia M. Donlen
Ruth A. Budd

The infant weighing less than 2500g at birth, generally referred to as a low-birth-weight (LBW) infant, presents a special challenge to nurses. Traditionally, nurses have been concerned with the health of their patients, the focus of nursing being to promote or maintain the patient's optimal health state. In the LBW infant, this optimal health state must be viewed in the context of either immaturity or deficient intrauterine growth. Such infants often require a great deal of support to maintain their optimal states. The nurse caring for the LBW infant uses the nursing process to assess, plan, and intervene to promote the best possible condition for the baby.

THEORETICAL FRAMEWORK

The LBW infant, like all human beings, is an interactive system; i.e., he responds to physiologic stressors as well as to those in his environment. The infant's adaptation to extrauterine life depends on his ability to cope with specific forces that act to disrupt his steady state. The neonatal nurse needs to view the baby in constant interaction with his environment and to plan nursing care to reduce the stressors that act to upset his equilibrium.

The types of interventions the nurse utilizes in caring for these infants have been described by Betty Neuman in her conceptual model.[1] In this scheme, the term primary prevention is used to designate actions that occur prior to the infant's encounter with the stressor. Secondary prevention refers to those interventions used to identify and reduce the early effects of the encountered stressor. Tertiary prevention describes actions that promote the restoration and maintenance of the infant's steady state after a period of disequilibrium. All of these nursing interventions are planned around the variables—physiologic, psychologic, sociocultural and developmental—that interact to give the composite picture of this small human being.

The physiologic focus of nursing care is on maintaining a neutral thermal environment and preserving the baby's energy stores while providing adequate nutrition. Other actions aim to counteract environmental and internal stressors that the baby is unable to handle because of organ and tissue dysmaturity.

The psychologic emphasis of nursing care is to provide a quiet and soothing environment for a baby whose condition may warrant many painful procedures. Stroking and other human contacts are aimed at reducing the impact of harmful forces.

In keeping with sociocultural considerations, the neonatal nurse involves the entire family in planning and implementing care for the LBW infant. Extended periods of private interaction help to balance the disequilibrium resulting from forced separation. Respect for cultural differences by the nursing staff also promotes family–infant bonds.

In response to developmental factors, nursing interventions are planned to encourage growth and development that are as close as possible to normal. Stimulation activities are planned as appropriate to expand the infant's auditory, visual, tactile, and kinesthetic senses.

CLASSIFICATION OF THE LBW INFANT

It has long been known that birth weight is important in predicting problems in newborn infants. Since birth weight and gestational age are interrelated, deviation in either weight or gestational age from the range considered to be physiologically normal results in increased neonatal morbidity. Gestational age may be calculated from the mother's last normal menstrual period, but often the dates are inaccurate because of postconceptual or irregular bleeding. Gestational age may also be clinically estimated after birth by assessing certain physical and neurologic criteria.

External or physical criteria useful in assessing gestational age include the presence of vernix caseosa, breast tissue development, shape and cartilage development of the ear, the depth of sole creases, skin texture and appearance, the presence of lanugo, the amount and texture of hair, genital development, and skull firmness. These criteria are best assessed within the first 24 hrs after birth. Two neurologic criteria are also assessed within the first day—resting posture and arm and leg recoil. Other neurologic criteria are most accurately assessed after the first 24 hrs, when the infant is in a quiet, rested state. These criteria include the heel-to-ear maneuver, scarf sign, the tone of the neck flexors and the neck and body extensors, vertical and horizontal positions of the body, flexion angles (popliteal, ankle, and square window), and primitive newborn reflexes.

Figure 1-1 delineates the expected maturation during gestation in terms of the physical and neurologic criteria described above. These criteria of maturation are independent of the amount of weight gained by the fetus. The neonatal nurse utilizes data collected on this scale to estimate the gestational age (weeks).

The infant's overall condition must be considered when a clinical assessment of gestational age is made. Not all criteria can be accurately assessed. Primitive newborn reflexes are often difficult to elicit, particularly in an already physiologically stressed newborn. Maneuvers involving active muscle tone, such as recoil or head lag seem to be a better indication of illness or well-being than of maturation. Physical criteria such as edema and skin color are inconsistently reliable depending on the clinical condition of the infant.

Certain criteria for assessing gestational age are less reliable when estimating the ages of infants of toxemic or diabetic mothers. Maternal toxemic states seem to accelerate fetal maturity while retarding fetal growth. Conversely, maternal diabetic states (Classes A through C) generally appear to accelerate fetal growth but retard maturity.

Once gestational age has been clinically assessed, the LBW infant can be classified according to growth in the following ways:

1. Term, small for gestational age (SGA)
2. Preterm, small for gestational age (SGA)
3. Preterm, appropriate for gestational age (AGA)
4. Preterm, large for gestational age (LGA)

The SGA, AGA, and LGA categories are determined by plotting the infant's birth weight and gestational age in weeks against a set standard for intrauterine growth (Fig. 1-2). The Colorado Intrauterine Growth Chart has been used widely throughout the United States for this purpose. When weights are plotted on this chart, infants whose weights fall below the 10th percentile are called undergrown (SGA); those whose weights fall between the 10th and 90th percentile are considered of appropriate weight (AGA); and those with weights above the 90th percentile are termed overgrown, (LGA).

Planning nursing care for the LBW infant begins with classifying the infant as preterm or term; and subsequently as SGA, AGA, or LGA. This classification scheme is the most useful tool for predicting problems related to gestational age and/or intrauterine growth. Once predicted, stressors can be decreased and supportive nursing care begun to facilitate the LBW infant's adaptation to his new environment. This is the level of care described above as "primary prevention."

Nurses can predict problems in preterm infants related to organ and tissue

Examination First Hours

WEEKS GESTATION

Week scale: 20 21 22 23 24 25 26 27 28 29 30 31 32 33 34 35 36 37 38 39 40 41 42 43 44 45 46 47 48

PHYSICAL FINDINGS		Findings (approximate week of appearance)
Vernix		Appears (21) · Covers body, thick layer (24–28) · On back, scalp, in creases (38) · Scant, in creases (40) · No vernix (42–44)
Breast tissue and areola		Areola and nipple barely visible, no palpable breast tissue (22–27) · Areola raised (34) · 1–2 mm nodule (36) · 3–5 mm (38) · 5–6 mm (39) · 7–10 mm (41) · ?12 mm (44)
Ear	Form	Flat, shapeless (21) · Beginning incurving superior (34) · Incurving upper 2/3 pinnae (37) · Well-defined incurving to lobe (40)
	Cartilage	Pinna soft, stays folded (22) · Cartilage scant, returns slowly from folding (33) · Thin cartilage, springs back from folding (37) · Pinna firm, remains erect from head (42)
Sole creases		Smooth soles without creases (22) · 1–2 anterior creases (35) · 2–3 anterior creases (35) · Creases anterior 2/3 sole (37) · Creases involving heel (41) · Deeper creases over entire sole (44)
Skin	Thickness & appearance	Thin, translucent skin, plethoric, venules over abdomen, edema (24–30) · Smooth, thicker, no edema (34) · Pink (37) · Some desquamation, pale pink (41) · Thick, pale, desquamation over entire body (44)
	Nail plates	Appear (23) · Nails to finger tips (34) · Nails extend well beyond finger tips (44)
Hair		Appears on head (23) · Eye brows and lashes (25) · Fine, woolly, bunches out from head (29) · Silky, single strands, lays flat (38) · ?Receding hairline or loss of baby hair, short, fine underneath (43)
Lanugo		Appears (21) · Covers entire body (23) · Vanishes from face (35) · Present on shoulders (41) · No lanugo (44)
Genitalia	Testes	Testes palpable in inguinal canal (29) · In upper scrotum (38) · In lower scrotum (42)
	Scrotum	Few rugae (29) · Rugae, anterior portion (37) · Rugae cover (40) · Pendulous (42)
	Labia & clitoris	Prominent clitoris, labia majora small, widely separated (30) · Labia majora larger, nearly cover clitoris (37) · Labia minora and clitoris covered (41)
Skull firmness		Bones are soft (22) · Soft to 1" from anterior fontanelle (29) · Spongy at edges of fontanelle, center firm (35) · Bones hard, sutures easily displaced (39) · Bones hard, cannot be displaced (44)
Posture	Resting	Hypotonic, lateral decubitus (21) · Hypotonic (27) · Beginning flexion, thigh (30) · Stronger hip flexion (32) · Frog-like (35) · Flexion, all limbs (37) · Hypertonic (39) · Very hypertonic (44)

Recoil - leg

	No recoil	Partial recoil	Prompt recoil
Arm	No recoil	Prompt recoil, may be inhibited	Prompt recoil after 30" inhibition

20	21	22	23	24	25	26	27	28	29	30	31	32	33	34	35	36	37	38	39	40	41	42	43	44	45	46	47	48

Begin flexion, no recoil

Confirmatory Neurologic Examination To Be Done After 24 Hours

Weeks Gestation

Physical Findings	20	21	22	23	24	25	26	27	28	29	30	31	32	33	34	35	36	37	38	39	40	41	42	43	44	45	46	47	48

Tone

- **Heel to ear:** No resistance | Some resistance | Impossible
- **Scarf sign:** No resistance | Elbow passes midline | Elbow at midline | Elbow does not reach midline
- **Neck flexors (head lag):** Absent | Head in plane of body | Holds head
- **Neck extensors:** Head begins to right itself from flexed position | Good righting cannot hold it | Holds head few seconds | Keeps head in line with trunk > 40" | Turns head from side to side
- **Body extensors:** Straightening of legs | Straightening of trunk | Straightening of head and trunk together
- **Vertical positions:** When held under arms, body slips through hands | Arms hold baby, legs extended? | Legs flexed, good support with arms
- **Horizontal positions:** Hypotonic, arms and legs straight | Arms and legs flexed | Head and back even, flexed extremities | Head above back

(Fig. 1-1. continues)

		20	21	22	23	24	25	26	27	28	29	30	31	32	33	34	35	36	37	38	39	40	41	42	43	44	45	46	47	48
Flexion angles	Popliteal	No resistance								150°				110°		100°				90°		80°								
	Ankle													45°				20°				0	A pre-term who has reached 40 weeks still has a 40° angle							
	Wrist (square window)									90°				60°				45°		30°		0								
Reflexes	Sucking							Weak, not synchronized with swallowing						Stronger, synchronized		Perfect				Perfect, hand to mouth				Perfect						
	Rooting							Long latency period slow, imperfect				Hand to mouth				Brisk, complete, durable								Complete						
	Grasp							Finger grasp is good, strength is poor						Stronger						Can lift baby off bed, involves arms								Hands open		
	Moro	Barely apparent						Weak, not elicited every time						Stronger		Complete with arm extension, open fingers, cry				Arm adduction added								?Begins to lose Moro		
	Crossed extension							Flexion and extension in a random, purposeless pattern						Extension, no adduction		Still incomplete				Extension, adduction, fanning of toes				Complete						
	Automatic walk											Minimal		Begins tiptoeing, good support on sole				Fast tiptoeing		Heel-toe progression, whole sole of foot				A pre-term who has reached 40 weeks walks on toes				?Begins to lose automatic walk		
	Pupillary reflex	Absent									Appears		Present																	
	Glabellar tap	Absent												Appears		Present														
	Tonic neck reflex	Absent								Appears				Present																
	Neck-righting	Absent														Appears			Present after 37 weeks											

Fig. 1-1. Clinical Estimation of Gestational Age. From Kempe CH, Silver HK and O'Brien D: Current Pediatric Diagnosis and Treatment, 3rd edition. Los Altos, Calif. Lange Medical Publications, 1974, pp 44–45

GRAMS

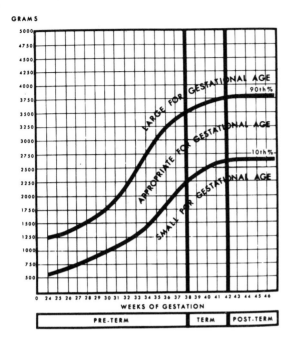

Fig. 1-2. Classification of Newborns by Birthweight and Gestational Age. From Battaglia, FC and Lubchenco, LO. J Pediat. 71:159, 1967

immaturity. Problems that should be anticipated in the premature AGA infant are different from those expected in the term or near-term SGA baby although their birth weights may be identical. The more premature the SGA baby, the more likely that problems resulting from immaturity will arise along with the problems related to intrauterine growth deficiency.

Pulmonary problems should be anticipated in both premature and SGA newborns; however, the premature AGA infant is at high risk for hyaline membrane disease (HMD), whereas the SGA baby is at risk for respiratory distress due to perinatal asphyxia—i.e., asphyxia resulting in aspiration of amniotic fluid and/or meconium or subsequent persistent pulmonary hypertension. Apnea is a common occurrence in the LBW infant, either because of prematurity or as a complication of perinatal asphyxia. Cardiac problems are somewhat unusual in preterm infants except for patent ductus arteriosus (PDA), which should be anticipated in preterm AGA infants, especially the more immature infants with HMD. Cardiac anomalies do occur in SGA and LGA preterm infants but are generally associated with other complex defects (see Chapter 3).

Premature infants are highly susceptible to postnatal infections as the result of their immature immune system, physical properties such as thin skin and fragile capillaries, and their need for intravenous therapy. In SGA newborns there is an increased incidence of congenital infections, particularly of viral origin. Therefore, until the screening tests are negative, pregnant women should avoid direct contact with these infants.

Metabolic problems should be anticipated in both premature and SGA

Table 1-1. Comparison of Problems of Premature vs. Small-for-Gestational-Age Infants

	Premature	SGA
Pulmonary	hyaline membrane disease apnea*	aspiration syndrome meconium aspiration persistent pulmonary hypertension apnea
Cardiac	patent ductus arteriosus associated with RDS	patent ductus arteriosus associated with complex cardiac defects and PFC that mimics a cardiac lesion
Immunologic	postnatal infection	congenital viral infection
Metabolic	hypoglycemia hypocalcemia hyperbilirubinemia*	hypoglycemia* hypocalcemia* hyperbilirubinemia
Leading cause of death	intraventricular hemorrhage	congenital malformations

* Higher incidence in this group

infants. Premature infants are at particular risk for hypoglycemia, hypocalcemia, and hyperbilirubinemia. Because of their immaturity, they are not able to mobilize their glycogen or calcium stores as readily as term infants. Premature babies may also have increased utilization of glucose and calcium because of the physiologic stress that results from respiratory distress syndrome (RDS), cold, or perinatal asphyxia. Unconjugated hyperbilirubinemia should be anticipated in premature infants because of delayed conjugation of bilirubin and higher bilirubin load.

The SGA infant should be observed for signs of hypoglycemia and hypocalcemia that result from deficient glycogen stores and a higher metabolic rate as compared with those in the premature infant. Hyperbilirubinemia should be anticipated as a result of congenital infection. Hyperbilirubinemia may also result from polycythemia, which commonly occurs in SGA infants as a result of intrauterine hypoxia. (See Chapter 4 for nutritional interventions aimed at preventing or correcting these metabolic problems.)

Congenital malformations are 20 times more frequent in SGA infants than in premature AGA babies. Consequently, the leading cause of death in the SGA baby is congenital malformation. Premature infants are more likely to die from intraventricular hemorrhage, associated with various factors related to their immaturity and/or therapy. Table 1-1 summarizes the problems of premature versus SGA infants.

MAINTENANCE OF THERMAL STABILITY

An appropriate thermal environment—one that maintains the infant's core temperature while minimizing oxygen consumption—is essential for the high-risk infant. Body temperature reflects the balance of heat loss and gain. The LBW infant loses heat quickly because of a large surface-to-weight ratio and the lack of subcutaneous fat. Heat loss may occur by conduction, convection, evaporation, or radiation. Sources of heat gain may be external or internal, i.e., produced by the infant. To compensate for cold stress, LBW and preterm infants produce and conserve heat. They produce heat by three mechanisms: increased metabolic activity, increased muscular activity, and brown-fat metabolism, a thermogenic process unique to infants. All three mechanisms increase oxygen consumption. Other effects occur. The additional metabolic and muscular activity results in more glucose utilization and caloric expenditure. The brown-adipose-tissue (BAT) metabolism releases fatty acids into the circulation.

When combined with heat conservation mechanisms such as peripheral vasoconstriction, increased heat production may maintain the infant's core temperature within a normal range. However, use of these defense mechanisms is physiologically costly and may result in the following problems. The increased oxygen consumption mentioned above can further upset the balance between oxygen requirement and oxygen availability that is already a problem in infants with cardiorespiratory disease. Furthermore, a PO_2 below 30 torr abolishes the metabolic response to cold.[2] The use of glucose for heat production can potentiate the risk of hypoglycemia, which can inhibit BAT catabolism and depress the metabolic rate.[2] The increased caloric expenditure may also limit the infant's growth potential. Anaerobic metabolism caused by peripheral vasoconstriction and fatty acids produced during BAT metabolism can result in acidosis. Acidosis, in turn, can cause or potentiate problems such as increased pulmonary vascular resistance leading to right-to-left shunting of blood and thus to hypoxemia. Acidosis also affects myocardial function, transmission of nerve impulses, and the affinity of bilirubin for brain tissue.

A thermal environment suitable for all infants does not exist. Also, it is important to note that a normal body temperature reading is not always an accurate indication of the baby's thermal state. A classic example is that despite significant cold stress, the axillary temperature may remain normal because of its proximity to areas of abundant BAT. Therefore, to insure thermal stability, the nurse should assess the infant as he interacts with his environment. Signs such as increased activity and restlessness may hallmark increased heat production in response to cold stress. Similarly, peripheral cyanosis, mottling, cool extremities, and diminished capillary filling may indicate attempts to conserve heat.

Another way to insure thermal stability is to take precautions to prevent unnecessary heat loss. Among many measures, drafts should be avoided by placing isolettes and radiant warmers away from air-conditioning ducts and by removing sources such as free-flowing oxygen from manual resuscitation bags. These bags are often inadvertently left "flowing" in the infant's bed or hung at his console but aimed at him when they are used for resuscitations, to counteract apneic attacks, and for chest physiotherapy. Assessment of the infant's thermal status requires a keen awareness of the infant and his environment.

Open bed warmers used in many neonatal intensive care units (NICUs) supply the infant with radiant heat to balance his heat losses. Although the baby's temperature is maintained by using a servo-control device, the LBW baby may not be in a neutral thermal state. Some studies have indicated increased oxygen consumption in infants nursed on a radiantly heated open bed.[3,4] Another problem associated with use of these units is the increased insensible water loss. Many studies are now being conducted to examine methods that maximize the effectiveness of the radiant heat gains by manipulating the infant's environment.

Two measures that may decrease the infant's convective and evaporative heat losses are using a plastic body hood or thin plastic blanket and providing extra humidity. Convectively heated incubators control the environment by reducing heat loss through convection and evaporation. However, the infant can still lose heat to the incubator wall through radiation. The clear sides and top of standard convective incubators are constructed as a single wall or layer similar to a single pane of glass. The temperature of this wall is influenced by the ambient temperature inside and outside the incubator. Thus the mean temperature of this wall is cooler than the incubator air temperature. The use of plastic hoods or blankets within the incubator is an attempt to minimize radiant heat loss within single-walled incubators. Therefore, many investigators are now examining the efficacy of double-walled incubators in decreasing radiant heat loss.

SUPPORTING THE HYPERBILIRUBINEMIC INFANT

By adult standards, every newborn is hyperbilirubinemic during the first week after birth. The mean serum bilirubin for fullterm infants on the 3rd postnatal day is 6mg%. This "physiologic" jaundice occurs during the transitional state of bilirubin metabolism as the neonate develops mechanisms to replace the placental clearance of bilirubin. As may be expected, the transition to efficient bilirubin clearance is prolonged in premature infants. This delay may be exaggerated in the sick preterm infant.

Unconjugated bilirubin (indirect-reacting) is the end product of the breakdown of heme, which is contained in both red blood cells and non-erythrocyte tissue. Unconjugated bilirubin is lipid (fat) soluble and therefore cannot be excreted in bile or through the kidneys. It is transported to the liver in plasma, bound to albumin, to undergo conversion to the nontoxic glucuronide form. If unconjugated bilirubin is not bound to albumin, it may easily deposit in brain tissue.

Conjugated bilirubin (direct-reacting) is a nontoxic water-soluble complex. Lipid-soluble bilirubin enters the hepatocyte by attaching to one of two acceptor proteins, labeled Y and Z. Once in the liver, the enzyme glucuronyltransferase facilitates the attachment of bilirubin to glucuronic acid. The conjugated bilirubin then moves through the biliary tree into the small bowel, where bacteria causes its conversion to non-reabsorbable urobilinogen. In this form, it is excreted in both the stool and urine. In summary, the conversion process changes non-excretable, lipid-soluble bilirubin to the excretable, water-soluble urobilinogen derivative.

The fetus produces bilirubin and is capable of conjugating it in utero. Only unconjugated bilirubin, however, can be excreted across the placenta. For this reason, an enzyme, beta glucuronidase, deconjugates the bilirubin when it reaches the fetal small bowel. This deconjugation process, which continues for some time after birth, is called the enterohepatic shunt and may be the most important cause of hyperbilirubinemia in the neonatal period. Other factors that contribute to hyperbilirubinemia in the LBW infant are as follows:

At birth, the premature neonate is less well prepared than the term infant to begin the process of conjugation because of a lower level of acceptor proteins and a less active glucuronyl transferase system. Moreover, the bilirubin load may be higher in premature neonates. These infants have a greater propensity for bleeding and hemolysis because of trauma during the perinatal period, and the percentage of shorter-lived fetal hemoglobin is higher. In addition, the enterohepatic shunt may be prolonged as the result of delayed feeding, which diminishes gastrointestinal motility and prevents bacterial colonization. This prolongation also increases serum levels of unconjugated bilirubin.

The premature infant is also more susceptible to the toxic effects of un-conjugated bilirubin, a specific neurotoxin that causes ballooning and degen-eration of neurons. There are several mechanisms for the susceptibility: levels of total protein and albumin are usually lower, so that more "free" bilirubin can enter the brain and cause bilirubin encephalopathy (kernicterus); fatty acids (produced during episodes of BAT thermogenesis or hypoglycemia) and certain drugs compete with bilirubin for albumin binding sites; and acidosis appears to increase the affinity of bilirubin for brain tissue. Bilirubin levels can only be considered safe within the context of the baby's perinatal experiences.

Phototherapy is often used to treat hyperbilirubinemia. A high-intensity light source is employed to deliver irradiation at an optimal wave length of 450 nanometers(nm). The dosage range for the intensity of this light is 4-14 μW/cm^2/nm; the dose depends on the rate of bilirubin production.[5,6] To prevent overexposure, a photometer is used at the infant's skin to measure the units of energy. Currently, it is thought that the beneficial effect of phototherapy results from photo-isomerization, rather than from photo-oxidation; i.e., the light transforms the bilirubin molecule into its isomer photobilirubin (bilirubin E), which is water-soluble. Bilirubin photoisomers that are water-soluble can be excreted directly in the urine or bile without undergoing conjugation.[7] Al-though a commonly used treatment modality, phototherapy is not without side effects. Recognition of this helps the nurse to plan nursing actions that prevent or diminish its undesirable effects on the infant.

Phototherapy is not without risk. Because retinal damage may result from the intense light, protective eye patches are needed during phototherapy. The baby's eyes should be closed before patches are applied. Care should also be taken to avoid a tight fit because the eye patches might obstruct the baby's airway. Patches that are too tight have also been implicated as a source of obstruction to cerebral venous blood return.[8] Phototherapy may also cause hyperthermia and increase insensible water loss. The use of servo-controlled incubators or warmers can eliminate the problem of over-heating. The in-creased fluid loss, although an anticipated side effect, is difficult to predict with accuracy. The smaller the infant, the more prone he is to potentially dangerous fluid imbalances. Weighing the infant every 8–12 hrs gives the most accurate information concerning the state of hydration.

Phototherapy often causes loose stools. This occurs because phototherapy increases gut motility, which then decreases gastrointestinal transit time. As food moves through at a faster rate, changes occur in the frequency, consistency, and color of stools, and increased stooling or diarrhea results. Bilirubin isomers may also affect the bowel to increase stooling. A further reason for increased gut irritability is that the activity of lactase, the enzyme that aids in the digestion of lactose, is often decreased in infants receiving phototherapy. This decreased activity may occur because the increased bile flow of unconjugated bilirubin—a non-specific effect of phototherapy—inhibits intestinal lactase secretion and therefore decreases the digestion of lactose. Thus, these infants have a limited ability to digest most of the commonly used formulas. The fluid loss accompanying such diarrhea can often further complicate the infant's precarious fluid balance. Substituting a formula with another carbohydrate source allows adequate nutrition and eliminates the problem of increased water loss through the gastrointestinal tract.

Early feeding of the premature infant can also help to reduce the peak bilirubin level. By supplying glucose and protein, feeding provides the substrates necessary for the albumin binding, transport, and conjugation of bilirubin. As mentioned above, feeding also decreases the enterohepatic shunt through bacterial colonization of the bowel and passage of stool.

SUPPORTING NEUROLOGIC INTEGRITY

Intraventricular hemorrhage (IVH) is one of the most feared complications in the LBW infant. Various studies have shown that, even though increasing numbers of premature infants survive the neonatal period, IVH is still a leading cause of death in this group. It is also responsible for moderate or severe neurological handicap in many survivors.[9]

The classical picture of the infant suffering an IVH is one of acute deterioration. The baby becomes ashen, hypotensive, hypotonic, and apneic. There may be generalized or focal seizures that are unresponsive to anticonvulsant therapy. The baby often develops temperature instability and may be unresponsive to stimuli. A drop in hematocrit and a persistent metabolic acidosis usually occur. Within a few hours, the anterior fontanel is bulging and taut. Death often occurs within hours of the onset of the symptoms. Recent studies, however, have pointed to the difficulty in correlating the occurrence of IVH with the classical signs and symptoms.[10] In infants with mild or moderate insults, the clinical picture is less definitive. Some infants may show subtle changes in color, tone, and responsiveness while vital signs remain unchanged. Other infants may never demonstrate observable symptoms.

Computerized tomography (CT) and ultrasound studies have yielded new information concerning the incidence of IVH in premature infants. Many hemorrhages that might otherwise be missed have been diagnosed by these studies. Although blood actually does enter the ventricles in 80% of the cases,[11] the term periventricular hemorrhage is probably a more accurate designation. The CT scan has also been useful, combined with postmortem data, in classifying the severity of the insult. The following classification scheme is used:[12]

Grade I, isolated subependymal hemorrhage;

Grade II, intraventricular hemorrhage without ventricular dilatation;

Grade III, intraventricular hemorrhage with ventricular dilatation;

Grade IV, intraventricular hemorrhage with ventricular hemorrhage and hemorrhage into the parenchyma of the brain.

This grading system seems to correlate with the infant's prognosis for survival, the likelihood that handicaps will occur, and the appearance of hydrocephalus.[9]

Recognition of the high incidence of periventricular hemorrhage in the preterm infant has led to an examination of the characteristics that might explain the phenomenon. The periventricular area is the site of the subependymal germinal matrix. This fetal structure is highly vascularized because of its role in forming cerebral glial cells during the 6th–8th months of gestation. The subependymal germinal matrix, no longer present in the term infant, offers poor support for its abundant capillary network in the premature infant. In addition, studies have shown increased fibrinolytic activity in the germinal matrix area of the immature brain, which may delay clotting should a bleeding episode occur.[13] The precipitating event in IVH seems to be related to the interaction of the large amount of blood in the germinal matrix with factors affecting the cerebral venous and arterial circulations.

Traditionally, the explanation for the often observed rupture of capillaries and small vessels in the periventricular area has been the occurrence of cerebral venous congestion. Venous blood draining from the periventricular area changes direction at a sharp angle as it joins with the internal cerebral vein. This change in the direction of flow would be expected to encourage venous stasis and congestion. Hypoxia and hypotension in the sick infant might precipitate circulatory failure and cerebral hypoperfusion. These conditions may lead to venous congestion and injury to the capillary wall, increasing the risk of rupture.[14] Recently, emphasis has shifted to arterial overperfusion as a possible cause of capillary rupture in the subependymal germinal matrix. Autoregulation, the ability to maintain the cerebral circulation pressure at safe levels through changes in cerebral vascular tone, is impaired in sick preterm infants.[15] The vasodilating effects of hypoxia and hypercapnea may allow the systemic pressure to be transmitted directly on the germinal matrix vascular bed, causing the rupture of these thin-walled, poorly supported capillaries.

Volume expansion during episodes of circulatory failure, hypernatremia, and hyperosmolarity have all been implicated in affecting both arterial and venous hemodynamics. Increased intrapleural pressure has also been associated with an increased incidence of IVH in the premature infant, presumably because it increases cerebral venous pressure. This effect is more likely to occur in mechanically ventilated infants whose lung compliance is good, such as those ventilated for apnea, since the positive pressure is more easily transmitted to the pleural space under these conditions. Similarly, the incidence of IVH is also increased in infants who develop a pneumothorax during mechanical ventilation.[16]

The mortality and neurologic sequelae associated with periventricular hemorrhage make its prevention—or at least limiting its extension—imperative. Identifying the infant at risk is the first step in planning nursing care. The more immature the infant, the more vulnerable he will be. The preterm infant who has been hypoxemic—either during birth or because of lung disease—should be considered at risk for loss of cerebral autoregulation. This would render cerebral blood flow dependent on the systemic blood pressure. The infant can suffer ischemic injury during periods of low blood flow, an event that increases the risk of a bleeding episode as the systemic blood pressure rises. Therefore, monitoring blood pressure is of critical importance. The amount of fluid administered and the urine output must be carefully observed to avoid either fluid depletion or fluid overload that could adversely affect systemic vascular pressure. The head-down position (such as that used in chest physiotherapy) may also be ill-advised, because of its potential effect on cerebral blood flow in the stressed preterm infant. The use of bicarbonate to correct metabolic acidosis can affect cerebral blood flow as well. The hyperosmolar nature of the solution may mobilize extravascular fluid and increase intravascular pressure. The transport of bicarbonate as dissolved carbon dioxide may transiently raise the PCO_2, dilating cerebral vessels. These effects warrant care during its administration. In addition to using at least a 1:1 dilution of $NaHCO_3$, the nurse must administer the correction dose over at least a 20–30 min interval.

Prevention of environmental stressors that may cause or potentiate hypoxemia should also be a prime objective of nursing care for these infants. Transcutaneous monitoring of oxygen can be helpful in determining the immediate effects of care on the infant's status. Clustering necessary nursing interventions helps to minimize excessive handling. Handling and the presence of irritating stimuli may be associated with decreased transcutaneous PO_2.[17] Handling may also raise the infant's systemic blood pressure. Each nursing action should be examined for its effect on the infant, modified to cause the least amount of stress, and prescribed for individual infants only when the benefit to be derived outweighs the risk. Weighing, suctioning, repositioning, and moving the infant for diagnostic procedures are examples of necessary actions that carry an increased risk for the stressed preterm infant. In general, an attitude of "watchful neglect" might best benefit these infants.

In addition to promoting thermal stability and adequate ventilation, oxygenation and perfusion, the nurse needs to provide a safe environment for the infant. External pressure exerted on the soft cranium of the preterm infant may have a role in the etiology of IVH by impeding cerebral blood flow.[18] This has implications for nurses caring for these infants. The avoidance of tight-fitting phototherapy masks and the use of a frame to support ventilator tubings may help to decrease the effect of external pressure on cerebral blood flow. Care must also be taken in the amount of pressure that is applied when using a face mask to ventilate a preterm infant. Water-filled mattresses may also diminish the effects of pressure on the infant's skull. Many routine practices will probably come under scrutiny in the near future, as the prevention of periventricular insult becomes a prime objective in the care of the high-risk infant.

THE LBW INFANT—A SOCIAL BEING

Infants, including those of LBW, are social interactive beings, capable of deriving pleasure from various verbal, tactile, auditory, and visual stimuli in their immediate environment. From the moment of birth, they respond to their extrauterine environment with various behaviors that are related to the state of consciousness. A reflection of the infant's potential for behavioral organization is his use of state of consciousness to react to various environmental and internal stressors. The six states of consciousness have been defined by Prechtl and Brazelton as deep sleep, light sleep, drowsy, quiet alert, active alert and crying.[19,20] The behavior exhibited by the infant depends on his state of consciousness when the stimulus was received.

From the first contact between parents and newborn, the parents observe their baby's behavior and use his appearance to form an image of who the baby is and how the baby feels about them. LBW infants demonstrate sleep patterns very different from those of term AGA infants. These smaller babies spend less time in the awake states, thereby decreasing parent–infant interaction time. As post-conceptional age increases, the ability to organize state develops.

Parent–infant attachment develops over a period of time through the process of reciprocal interactions. Parents elicit behaviors in their newborn that are pleasing to them. Infants also elicit behaviors in their parents. These infant behaviors, termed by Bowlby "releasers of maternal caretaking responses," include crying, smiling, following, clinging, sucking, and eye-to-eye contact.[21] However, the LBW infant demonstrates few of these behaviors because of his immaturity and/or CNS disorganization from deficiency in intrauterine growth. "Primary prevention" of disturbed parent–child relationships begins here. When the infant cannot be held, the nurse working with the parents can encourage them to speak to their infant, look at his face, and gently touch and stroke him. When the infant is stable enough to be held despite the need for mechanical ventilation and other supportive measures, the nurse can encourage them also to cuddle their infant face to face in a rocking chair. She can teach parents about infant behaviors and capabilities, thus further encouraging interaction.

The cognitive development of LBW infants has been related to variables such as the degree of prematurity and of morbidity and the effectiveness of parent–infant interaction.[22] The latter, however, is jeopardized by the NICU environment. Barriers such as equipment necessary for physiologic support of the infant often restrict the parent–infant acquaintance process. Additional limitations to early contact are treatment regimens such as prolonged phototherapy, intravenous therapy and mechanical ventilation.

Other inhibitors of normal development are commonly present in the NICU environment. LBW infants are exposed to noise from incubator motors, airflow, ventilators, chest-tube suction apparatus and talking. It has been suggested that incubators impede language development by masking, attenuating, or distorting sounds.[23] In adults, the maximum sound intensity that can be endured without producing sensorineural hearing loss is 80 decibels (db). The American Academy of Pediatrics recommends that NICU noise levels be kept to below 75 db.[23] However, a survey of NICUs revealed a normal range of 80–100 db. Potentiation of noise-induced hearing loss to as much as 100-fold by the ototoxic aminoglycosidic antibiotics has been established in animal studies.[23] Kanamycin and neomycin seem to have the greatest potentiating effects; streptomycin, gentamycin and tobramycin still require further study. Particularly when caring for LBW infants who are being treated with aminoglycocides, nurses must make every effort to reduce the noise levels to within an acceptable range.

The use of constant daylight in the NICU environment must also be considered an inhibitor to normal development. Studies have shown that infants exposed to constant daylight for the first few weeks of life have difficulty establishing a regular sleeping pattern at home.[24] Another area of concern is that infants in the NICU often lack appropriate visual stimulation. Term newborns are capable of fixating on bright objects within a distance of 7–9 inches. The LBW infant should have bright objects such as checkerboard or stabile face patterns placed within 7–9 inches of his face to encourage visual fixation. Parents should also be encouraged to establish eye-to-eye contact with their infants.

Appropriate tactile stimulation may be lacking for the LBW infant. The baby's condition often requires many painful treatments or procedures. Planned, sustained stimulation activities such as stroking or holding "en face" have been shown to increase developmental scores in the LBW infant.[25] Programs such as those described in the Education for Multihandicapped Infants (EMI) High Risk Nursery Intervention Program[26] and the Portage Guide to Early Education[27] are easily implemented in the NICU. The stimulation programs are developed to include parents in planning and implementing specific interventions for their infants. Thus, a strong foundation is set for continued positive parent–child interaction following discharge from the unit.

One of the features of effective mother–infant interaction is the mother's sensitivity to her infant's behaviors. Nurses need to become expert observers of infant behavioral organization and to identify the environmental variables that enhance and sabotage infant behavior.[28] Nurses must then interpret this information for the parents to teach them what soothes and what irritates their infant.

Recent research has suggested that the Brazelton Neonatal Behavioral Assessment Scale (BNBAS) is a useful intervention tool to be used by nurses in teaching parents about the behavior patterns of their newborns.[22] This tool provides the nurse and family with a wealth of information that includes individual behavioral characteristics of that infant, level of neurologic function, and capacity to interact with his environment.[29] Use of an adaptation of the BNBAS, termed as the Mother's Assessment of the Behavior of Her Infant Scale (MABI) indicated that mothers of healthy preterm infants who assessed their own infants weekly, appeared to interact more effectively with their babies. As compared with a control group of preterm infants whose mothers did not administer the scale, these experimental group infants demonstrated higher Bayley Scales scores at one year.[30] By focusing on a wide range of newborn behavioral characteristics and interactive capabilities, nurses caring for LBW infants and their families can facilitate effective parent–infant interaction and subsequent social and psychological development of the infant.

CONCLUSION

The LBW infant is at risk, from the moment of his birth, for many problems related to his immaturity and to the events occurring during his perinatal course. Improvements in medical care have enabled many of these infants to survive, but the quality of their survival can depend on the nursing care they receive during their neonatal period. As research yields new information concerning the physiology of the preterm infant and his interaction with his environment, new treatment modalities will be developed. The nurse caring for the LBW infant needs to examine nursing care procedures in light of this developing knowledge base. The goal of improving perinatal outcome necessitates a team approach that assures the best possible health state for every infant.

REFERENCES

1. Neuman B: The Betty Neuman health-care systems model: a total person approach to patient problems. In: Conceptual Models for Nursing Practice. 2nd edn. eds. Riehl JP and Roy C New York, Appleton-Century-Crofts, 1980, pp 119–134
2. Davis V: The structure and function of brown adipose tissue in the neonate. JOGN Nurs 9:371, 1980, pp 368–372
3. LeBlanc MH: The relative efficacy of an incubator in producing thermoneutrality in small prematures. Pediatr Res 15:669, 1981 (abstract)
4. Gerhardt T, Feller R, Bancalari E: Increased O_2 consumption in premature infants under radiant warmers. Pediatr Res 14:598, 1981 (abstract)
5. Korones SB: Neonatal Jaundice. In: High-Risk Newborn Infants: The Basis for Intensive Care Nursing. 3rd ed. St. Louis, CV Mosby, 1981, pp 285–300
6. Tan KL: Comparison of the effectiveness of single-direction and double-direction phototherapy for neonatal jaundice. Pediatrics 56:550–553, 1975
7. Bakken AF: Temporary intestinal lactase deficiency in light-heated jaundiced infants. Acta Paediatr Scand 66:91, 1977

8. Kosmetatos N, Williams ML: Effect of positioning and head banding on intracranial pressure in the premature infant. Pediatr Res 12:553, 1978 (abstract)
9. Korones SB: Central nervous system disorders of perinatal origin. In: High Risk Newborn Infants: the Basis for Intensive Nursing Care. 3rd ed. St Louis, CV Mosby, 1981, pp 342–353
10. Lazzara A, Ahmann P, Dykes F, et al.: Clinical predictability of intraventricular hemorrhage in preterm infants. Pediatrics 65:30–34, 1980
11. Volpe JJ: Intracranial hemorrhage in the newborn: current understanding and dilemmas. Neurology 29:632–635, 1979
12. Fenichel GM: Neonatal Neurology. New York, Churchill Livingstone, 1980, pp 94
13. Price FH, Kezy SV, Berenberg W: Fibrinolytic activity in the ganglionic eminence of the premature human brain. Biol Neonate 18:426–432, 1971
14. Volpe JJ: Neonatal periventricular hemorrhage: past, present, and future. J Pediatr 92:693–696, 1978
15. Lou HC, Lassen NA, Fris-Hansen B: Impaired autoregulation of cerebral blood flow in the distressed newborn infant. J Pediatr 94:118, 1979
16. Dykes FD, Lazzara A, Ahmann P, et al.: Intraventricular hemorrhage: a prospective evaluation of etiopathogenesis. Pediatrics 66:42, 1980
17. Speidel BD: Adverse effects of routine procedures on preterm infants. Lancet 1:864, 1978
18. Pape KE, Wigglesworth JS: Haemorrhage, Ischaemia and the Perinatal Brain. Philadelphia, JB Lippincott, 1979
19. Prechtl HFR, Deintema O: Neurological Examination of the Fullterm Infant. London, Heinemann, 1964
20. Brazelton TB: Neonatal Behavioral Assessment Scale. Philadelphia, J.B. Lippincott, 1973
21. Bowlby J: Attachment and Loss; Vol 1, Attachment. New York, Basic Books, 1973
22. Widmayer S, Field TM: Effects of Brazelton demonstrations for mothers on the development of preterm infants. Pediatrics 76:711–714, 1981
23. American Academy of Pediatrics Committee on Environmental Hazards: Noise pollution: neonatal aspects. Pediatrics 54:478, 1974
24. Desmond M, Wilson GS, Alt EJ, Fisher ES: The very low birth weight infant after discharge from intensive care: anticipatory health care and development course. In: Current Problems in Pediatrics. Chicago, Year Book Med Pub, Vol. 10, No. 6, 1980, p 13
25. Barnard KE: A Program of stimulation for infants born prematurely. Paper presented at the meetings of the Society for Research in Child Development, Philadelphia, April, 1973
26. Wallens P, Edler WB, Hastings SN: The EMI High Risk Nursery Intervention Program Manual. Charlottesville, University of Virginia Medical Center, 1979
27. Bluma S, Shearer M, Frohman A, Hilliard J: Portage Guide to Early Education. Portage, WI, Portage Project, 1976
28. Cooper BM, Schraeder BD: Developmental trends and behavioral styles in very low birth weight infants. Nurs Res 31:68, 1982
29. Brazelton TB: Neonatal Behavioral Assessment Scale. Philadelphia, JB Lippincott, 1973, p 4
30. Gibes RM: Clinical uses of the Brazelton Neonatal Behavioral Assessment Scale in nursing practice. Pediatr Nurs:23–26, 1981, p 23

SUGGESTED READINGS

Avery GB (ed): Neonatology. Philadelphia, JB Lippincott, 1981

Ballard JL, Novak KK, Driver M: A simplified score for assessment of fetal maturation of newly born infants. J Pediatr 95:769–774, 1979

Baumgart S, Engle WD, Fox WW, Polin RA: Environmental intervention and insensible water loss in critically ill neonates nursed under radiant warmers. Pediatr Res 14:590, 1980

Behrman RE: Neonatal-Perinatal Medicine. St Louis, CV Mosby, 1977

Bejar R, Curbelo V, Coen RW, Leopold G, James H, Gluck L: Diagnosis and follow-up of intraventricular and intracerebral hemorrhages by ultrasound studies of infant's brain through the fontanelles and sutures. Pediatrics 66:661, 1980

Brodersen R: Bilirubin transport in the newborn infant, reviewed with relation to kernicterus. J Pediatr 96: 349–356, 1980

Cole VA, Durbin GM, Olaffson A, et al.: Pathogenesis of intraventricular hemorrhage in newborn infants. Arch Dis Child, 49:722–728, 1974

Dubowitz LMS, Dubowitz V, Goldberg C: Clinical assessment of gestational age in the newborn infant. J Pediatr 77:1–10, 1970.

Endo AS: Using computers in newborn intensive care settings. AJN, 81: 1336–1337, 1981

Evaluation: Infant radiant warmers. Health Devices, 4: 128–142, 1975

Evaluation: Freestanding phototherapy units. Health Devices, 10 Nos. 6–7: 133–151, April-May, 1981

Field TM, Dempsey JR, Hallock NH, Shuman HH: The mother's assessment of the behavior of her infant. Infant Behavior and Development 1:156–167, 1978

Fitch CW, Korones SB, Wade JE: Measured reduction of radiant energy requirements in special heat shield. Pediatr Res 14:497, 1980

Gartner LM, Arias IM: Formation, transport and excretion of bilirubin. N Engl J Med 280:1339, 1969

Gerhardt T, Feller R, Bancalari E: Increased oxygen consumption in premature infants under radiant warmers. Pediatr Res 14:598, 1981

Hambleton G, Wigglesworth JS: Origin of intraventricular hemorrhage in the preterm infant. Arch Dis Child, 51:651–659, 1976

Klaus MH, Kennell JH: Maternal-Infant Bonding. St Louis, CV Mosby, 1976

Klaus M, Fanaroff A (eds): Care of the High Risk Neonate. Philadelphia, WB Saunders, 1980

Lou HC, Skov H, Pederson H: Low cerebral blood flow: a risk factor in the neonate. J Pediatr 95:606, 1979

Lubchenco LO: The High Risk Infant. Philadelphia, WB Saunders, 1976

Matheny AP: Assessment of infant mental development: Tetchy and Wayward approaches. Clin Perinatol 4:187–200, 1977

Nugent JK: The Brazelton Neonatal Behavioral Assessment Scale: implications for intervention. Pediatr Nurs: 18–21, 1981

Odell GB: Neonatal Hyperbilirubinemia. New York, Grune and Stratton, 1980

Papile L, Burstein J, Burstein R, Koffler H: Incidence and evolution of subendymal and intraventricular hemorrhage: a study of infants with birth weights less than 1500 gm. J Pediatr 92:529–534, 1978

Poland RL, Odell GB: Physiologic jaundice: the enterohepatic circulation of bilirubin. N Engl J Med 284:1, 1971

Riehl JP, Roy C (eds.): Conceptual models for nursing practice, 2nd edn, New York, Appleton-Century-Croft, 1981

Rogers MC, Nugent SK, Traystman RJ: Control of cerebral circulation in the neonate and infant. Crit Care Med 8:570–574, 1980

Stern L: Thermal environment of the newborn infant. Current Problems in Pediatrics 1:3, 1970

Volpe JJ: Current concepts in neonatal medicine: neonatal intraventricular hemorrhage. N Engl J Med 304:886, 1981

Volpe JJ: Neonatal intracranial hemorrhage. Clin Perinatol 4:77–102, 1977

White PL, Fomufod AK, Rao MS: Comparative accuracy of recent abbreviated methods of gestational age determination. Clin Pediatr 19:319–321, 1980

2 | Neonatal Mechanical Ventilation: Current Practice and Future Trends

Philip A. Balderston

High risk infants who develop acute respiratory failure and require ventilatory support for their survival have always presented a complex challenge to those who take care of them. In 1953, prior to the existence of neonatal intensive care units, Donald and Lord described the use of a patient-cycled, servocontrolled respirator in the treatment of several newborns exhibiting signs of respiratory distress.[1] Since then, significant advances have occurred in the technology and methods employed for mechanical ventilation of the neonate. Further, the types and qualifications of persons who take care of neonates have also changed to complement this process. The focus of this chapter is twofold; it presents: (1) current concepts and potential future trends in neonatal mechanical ventilation and (2) clinical application of physiologic and technologic concepts.

HISTORICAL PERSPECTIVE

Therapeutic and Technological Advances

Much has been accomplished in the relatively short period of time since Donald and Lord's work in 1953. During the 1950's, neonatal respiratory distress syndrome (RDS) was recognized as a phenomenon resulting from lung immaturity. In the early 1960's, the focus of national attention on the death of President Kennedy's son, born prematurely with RDS, spurred increasing interest in the treatment of the neonate in respiratory distress. The use of positive and negative pressure ventilators became accepted practice during the latter portion of this decade and their application continued to be refined during the early 1970's.

The decade of the 1970's was a time of great advances in the treatment of neonatal pulmonary disease. In 1971, Gregory et al described the use of continuous positive airway pressure (CPAP), a technique used successfully in the treatment of adult pulmonary disease, for the treatment of neonates with RDS.[2] Concurrently, continuous negative pressure (CNP) was reported as another method of providing continuous distending pressure for RDS.[3] When applied early, the use of these techniques has reduced the number of infants requiring mechanical ventilation.[4] Intermittent mandatory ventilation (IMV) was first introduced in the early 1970's as a technique for weaning patients from mechanical ventilation.[5] In the mid-1970's this technique gained wide acceptance in neonatal centers and IMV was incorporated into the design of many newly introduced neonatal mechanical ventilators. In 1978, Peckham and Fox advocated a new ventilatory technique in the treatment of persistent pulmonary hypertension of the neonate (PPHN)[6] that has led to the development of a new generation of mechanical ventilators with expanded rate capabilities.

Technologic advances paralleled the therapeutic advances of this decade with the development of sophisticated monitoring devices that yielded information previously unavailable or extremely difficult to obtain. Bedside devices that continuously measure and record variables such as transcutaneous levels of oxygen and carbon dioxide, the partial pressure of oxygen or the oxygen saturation of umbilical artery blood, or the pressures required for mechanical ventilation have contributed to the care of the neonate in this decade (see Adjunctive Monitoring). These contributions are a direct result of advances in electronics and computer technology.

Evolution of the Neonatal Care Environment

Prior to the mid-1960's, critically ill neonates were often cared for by physician and nursing staffs that were specially trained in adult life support techniques. The equipment available to provide the necessary support was not designed for neonatal application and attempts to "scale-down" this equipment often failed miserably. The inappropriateness of the available equipment was particularly evident in the area of mechanical ventilatory support. These factors contributed to an already poor prognosis for an infant born with significant respiratory distress.

The increasing interest in the underlying causes and treatment of neonatal pulmonary disease seen in the mid-1960's was accompanied by the establishment of specialized units to care for these infants. The designation of regional neonatal intensive care units in the 1970's, the majority of which occurred in university settings, resulted in a dramatic increase in the survival of very small infants.

Evolution of Neonatal Care Personnel

The regionalization of neonatal intensive care units further altered the approach to the care of critically ill neonates. The roles of physicians, nurses, and respiratory therapists have developed according to the needs placed on each group by scientific and technologic advances and regionalization of care. Although significant differences continue to exist, the level of practice and the types of practitioners found in neonatal care settings is determined by where a particular institution fits into this regional scheme.

The physician continues to be responsible for the medical direction of care for the mechanically ventilated neonate. However, factors such as the neonate's uniqueness and complexity in addition to those previously mentioned have created the need for the pediatric subspecialty of neonatology. In most level III centers, the neonatologist is responsible for the medical direction of mechanical ventilation in the treatment of neonatal pulmonary disease.

The critical care nursing role in neonatal intensive care has developed along with the increasing need for specialized care. This need is associated with the increased survival of very-low-birth-weight infants; this increased survival is due to the unprecedented research efforts and subspecialty groups interested in this population. While infants weighing less than 1500 grams were once thought too small to survive extrauterine life, today, infants above 700 grams are considered potentially viable. Caring for these neonates has created different expectations for the nurse, requiring additional knowledge of the very-low-birth-weight infant, refinement of clinical skills, and working with technology designed for use with this size newborn. Care that is considered routine and nonstressful in the older and larger newborn is very stressful for this group. Therefore, the nurse must be continually involved in the following areas: (1) evaluating the infant from a total perspective consisting of his degree of immaturity, growth and development, adaptation to stress, and response to therapy; and (2) interpreting, reporting, and integrating this knowledge with other disciplines to either minimize stressors or provide prompt and appropriate interventions.

The role of a respiratory therapy service in neonatal intensive care has changed significantly from that of a delivery service for respiratory equipment as existed in the 1960's. This has occurred primarily because of the need for a specialty group trained in the technical aspects and clinical application of the numerous, ongoing technologic and therapeutic advances. In many neonatal centers, respiratory therapists participate in the bedside care and assessment of the mechanically ventilated neonate. Also, the respiratory therapist's training in pulmonary physiology and its application to neonatal pulmonary disease provide the nursing and resident physician staffs with a strong educational resource.

NEONATAL PULMONARY PHYSIOLOGY: SOME BASIC CONCEPTS

Mechanical ventilation of the neonate differs radically from that of a child or an adult due to the uniqueness of neonatal pulmonary physiology. Therefore, to understand the rationales and controversies associated with the current state of the art, a sound knowledge of important neonatal pulmonary physiologic concepts is necessary.

Terminology

A review of some key terms that apply to pulmonary physiology will complement the later, more thorough discussion of physiologic concepts. These terms describe lung volumes and mechanical properties of the lungs as they relate specifically to the neonatal pulmonary system.

Lung Volumes   Four terms describe the volume of gas within the pulmonary system during a particular portion of the ventilatory cycle and are especially significant when discussing neonatal pulmonary physiology. These terms are: (1) tidal volume (V_t), (2) functional residual capacity (FRC), (3) expiratory reserve volume (ERV), and (4) residual volume (RV). Tidal volume is the volume of air that is inspired or exhaled with a single breath.

From the time a newborn takes his first breath a certain volume of air remains within the lungs following exhalation. This volume is created by the opposition of the retractive forces of the lung parenchyma and the expansive forces of the chest wall. These forces reach equilibrium at the end of exhalation (Fig. 2-1). The volume of air remaining at equilibrium is the FRC or resting volume of the lung. This volume remains constant with normal breathing.

The FRC is made up of two components. The ERV is that portion of the FRC that can be forced out with a maximal exhalation. This volume can be thought of as a reserve that may be called upon when the body is stressed and needs to increase pulmonary gas exchange. The second component or RV, is the volume of air that remains in the lungs. In neonates, the RV may be thought of as the collapse volume since as this volume is approached, an increasing proportion of alveoli collapse. The interrelationships of these lung volumes is shown in Figure 2-2.

Mechanical Properties of the Lung   Lung mechanics describe the relationship between pressure, volume and flow. Some mechanical properties of the lung are compliance, resistance and elastance. Of these, compliance and resistance are the most significant when managing neonatal pulmonary disease.

Compliance is a relationship between volume and pressure—the change in volume for a given pressure change. It is a measure of the expansibility of the lungs and/or thorax. Compliance can be thought of as an indication of the relative stiffness of the lungs. A decrease in lung compliance indicates an increase in stiffness or abnormal lung tissue and contributes significantly to the work of breathing in sick neonates. Lung compliance is most affected by

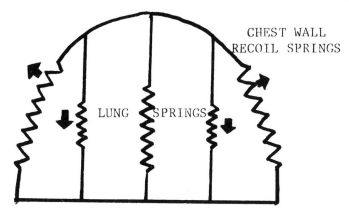

Fig. 2-1. Opposing forces of chest wall vs. lung elastic recoil. The position (and volume) of the thorax and lungs at end-expiration is where the forces balance out and where intrathoracic and airway pressures are equal. This is FRC or rest volume. (Harris TR: Physiological principles. In: Assisted Ventilation of the Neonate. ed. Goldsmith JP, Karotkin EH. Philadelphia, W.B. Saunders, 1981.)

factors that impair surfactant production, result in barotrauma, or lead to an accumulation of excess lung water.

Airway resistance, another mechanical property of the lung, is a relationship between pressure and flow—the change in pressure for a given flow. It is a measure of the difficulty of moving air through the conducting pathways on inspiration and expiration, and when increased, contributes to the work of

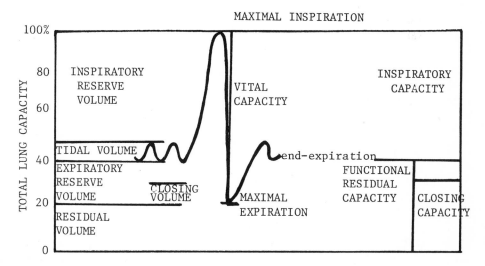

Fig. 2-2. Static lung volumes defined. A standard spirogram is shown for reference. (Smith CA, Nelson NM: Physiology of the Newborn Infant, 4th ed. Springfield, Charles C Thomas, 1976.)

EXAMPLE OF MEAN AIRWAY PRESSURE CALCULATION

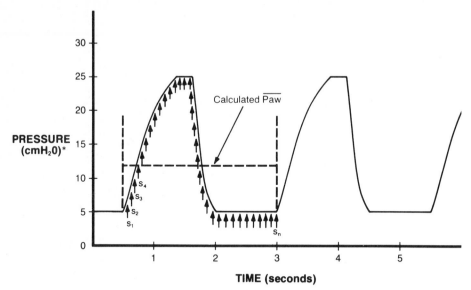

TIME (seconds)

Fig. 2-3.   A pressure-time trace showing calculation of mean airway pressure. (courtesy of Novametrix Medical Systems, Inc. Wallingford, Ct.). s_{1-4}, s_n = sample points q10 msec in microprocessor; $\overline{Paw}$ = MAP.

breathing. Airway resistance results from friction between molecules of flowing gas and the walls of airways as well as from viscous or frictional resistance of lung tissue. Its role in neonatal pulmonary disease is only in those processes where airway obstruction is the primary feature such as that seen in meconium aspiration syndrome when air trapping results in an increased A/P diameter. In most neonates who require mechanical ventilation, airway resistance is usually close to normal. However, this resistance can be increased in these infants if the airways are compromised such as with excess or dried secretions in their endotracheal tubes. When these infants are extubated, careful assessment is essential to evaluate for potential edema resulting from the nasotracheal or orotracheal tube. Edema of the nares may compromise the airway in the obligate nose breathing neonate. This is especially significant when a nasogastric tube is in place and/or periodic suction is necessary. Edema of the laryngopharynx may be more common and is often associated with stridor.

Two other terms that reflect both the clinical status of compliance and resistance and are affected by many of the physiologic concepts discussed in this section warrant definition here. Mean airway pressure (MAP) is a measure of the mean pressure applied to the neonatal pulmonary system during a ventilatory cycle. It can be described by looking at a tracing of a positive pressure breath (Fig. 2-3) and is affected by the ventilatory parameters in Table 2-7. The second term, transpulmonary pressure (TPP), is the difference between MAP and mean esophageal pressure and is a measure of the amount of pressure applied to the neonatal airways that is transmitted to the pleura. Since the esophageal pressure (measured by a balloon catheter) is an estimate of this pleural pressure, the difference between MAP and esophageal pressure is the amount of transmitted pressure.

Neonatal Lung Fragility

Important structural differences contrast the neonatal and adult pulmonary systems. The concept of neonatal lung fragility illustrates these differences by incorporating three elements: (1) chest wall instability; (2) fewer alveoli; and (3) lack of or impaired production of pulmonary surfactant.

The neonate's chest wall is almost infinitely distensible compared to the rigid chest wall structure of the adult. This is due to the lack of bony ossification and muscular development in the neonatal chest wall. The lack of rigidity reduces the expansive force generated by the chest wall or allows the chest wall to retract when increased negative pressure is generated. The lack of rigidity also allows the retractive force of the lung tissue to play a larger role in determining or reducing the FRC. This combination leads to a reduced

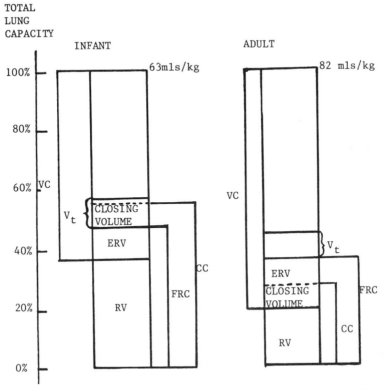

Fig. 2-4. Static lung volumes of the infant and adult. (Smith CA, Nelson NM: Physiology of the Newborn Infant. 4th ed. Springfield, Charles C Thomas, 1976)

Table 2-1. Alveolar Counts

Age Group	Estimated number of Alveoli for Terminal Lung Unit
Gestational Period	
24–27 weeks	42
32–35 weeks	130
Birth: 40 weeks	340
1 year	1370
2–3 years	1556
4–5 years	1715
7–8 years	2200
9–10 years	2630
11–12 years	3200

Adapted from: Emery JL, Mitwal A: The number of alveoli in the terminal respiratory unit in man during late intrauterine life and childhood. Arch Dis Child 35:544, 1960

expansive effect on the alveoli, decreased alveolar volume, and a proportional decrease in the neonate's FRC. Since the RV is fixed, the reduction in FRC is directly related to a fall in ERV. Therefore, the neonate breathes in a range of volume much closer to his RV. (Fig. 2-4). The stressed neonate's reserve volume is much smaller; this makes him more susceptible to early respiratory failure. Sternal and intercostal retractions secondary to decreased lung compliance factors are among the early signs and symptoms of respiratory distress in the neonate.

The second element contributing to lung fragility is fewer alveoli. The term infant has 10 percent of the number of alveoli that he will have as an adult. The preterm infant is further disadvantaged since his number of alveoli is proportionally less for each period of gestational age (Table 2-1).[7]

The third element contributing to lung fragility is a reduced amount of pulmonary surfactant present in premature infant lungs. This may lead to alveolar instability and atelectasis often seen in the preterm neonate requiring mechanical ventilation.

The combination of these three elements, called lung fragility, make the neonate's pulmonary mechanics and lung structure a remarkably different problem from the child's or adult's. Therefore, management of the preterm infant's respiratory problems can be a special challenge for the neonatal practitioner.

Surface Tension and Pulmonary Surfactant

In contrast to the adult, the major factor contributing to the retractive forces or elastic recoil of the neonatal lungs is surface tension at the air-alveolar interface.[8] La Place's law describes the amount of pressure necessary to overcome the tendency for alveoli to collapse by the formula:

$$P = 2 \, ST/r$$

where ST is the surface tension, r is the radius of the alveoli, and P is the pressure.

The radius of the alveolus is inversely related to the surface tension. Therefore, the smaller the radius, the greater the surface tension tending to cause alveolar collapse.

Surface tension at the air-alveolar interface is largely determined by the presence of sufficient amounts of pulmonary surfactant. This substance is a phospholipid monolayer that has the detergent or wetting agent property of varying surface tension with alveolar volume; that is, it enables surface tension to decrease as alveolar volume decreases during expiration. Therefore, it has a direct effect on the amount of pressure required to maintain a stable alveolar volume. Reduced amounts of surfactant make lung expansion more difficult and requires greater pressure to overcome the increased surface tension. Pulmonary surfactant decreases work of breathing, permits alveoli to remain inflated at low distending pressures, and reduces net forces causing tissue fluid accumulation.[9]

These factors combine in pulmonary disease seen in neonates born prematurely. Pulmonary surfactant develops late in gestation, appearing first at 28–30 weeks in an immature form, and its production is easily interrupted by factors such as hypoxia and acidosis. This leads to insufficient quantities available in the premature neonate. Also, the radius of alveoli in these neonates is inherently smaller when compared to that of a term infant. Hence, the premature infant is prone to alveolar collapse and the generation of large intrapulmonary pressures is often necessary to reopen these collapsed alveoli.

Lung compliance provides a measure of alveolar collapse and is often extremely poor in the premature infant. Poor compliance is particularly evident clinically when manually ventilating an infant with RDS compared to an infant without compliance disease. The infant with RDS will require more pressure or a "harder squeeze of the bag" to generate the same amount of chest wall movement. This increased inflating pressure, required with poor compliance, can be quantified by attaching a manometer to a resuscitation bag.

Intrapulmonary Shunting

A consequence of alveolar collapse described earlier was a fall in compliance. A second consequence seen in neonates in respiratory distress is an increase in intrapulmonary shunting when an increasing proportion of the blood perfusing the pulmonary capillary bed returns to the heart not having participated in gas exchange. This leads to hypoxemia which directly affects the pulmonary blood vessels by vasoconstriction, and results in an increase in pulmonary vascular resistance, reduced pulmonary blood flow, increased right-to-left intracardiac shunting, and further hypoxemia. The circular nature of this cycle causes the quick and severe deterioration seen in neonates with RDS when intervention is delayed.

NEONATAL MECHANICAL VENTILATION

The primary goal of neonatal mechanical ventilation is to maintain optimal gas exchange while causing the least amount of trauma to the fragile newborn pulmonary system. Adequate oxygenation and minimization of barotrauma allow normal tissue function and prevent lactic acidosis, shock, and right-to-left shunting. This goal illustrates the supportive nature of mechanical ventilation; neonatal mechanical ventilation does not provide a cure for the underlying pulmonary disease process.

The indications for instituting mechanical ventilatory support fall into two main categories: apnea and severe derangement of gas exchange.[10] Primary apnea or apnea from birth is an undisputable indication for mechanical ventilation but recurrent apneic periods may also result in the need for ventilatory support. These periods of apnea are often accompanied by a sudden decrease in heart rate and when an arterial blood sample is obtained, evidence of serious hypoxemia (PaO_2 less than 35 mm Hg) and frequently hypercapnia and acidemia are found.[10]

Derangements in pulmonary gas exchange are less clear-cut indications and depend on the perinatal course, gestational age, and age at the time of the blood gas sample. Table 2 illustrates a scoring system (based on arterial blood gas analysis) used to determine which infants require ventilatory assistance via CPAP therapy or mechanical ventilation.[11] The indications for mechanical ventilatory support are: (1) a score of 3 or greater; or (2) a partial pressure of oxygen in arterial blood (PaO_2) below 50 mm Hg in a fractional inspired oxygen concentration (FiO_2) of 0.6; or (3) CPAP failure defined as CPAP of 10 cm H_2O and an FiO_2 of 1.0. This scoring system is presented as an example; the need for ventilatory assistance as determined by arterial blood gas values may differ among neonatal centers. Factors such as transport time, delay in intervention, maternal history, along with those mentioned earlier, contribute to institutional criteria for mechanical ventilation.

Classification of Ventilators

Practitioners caring for critically ill neonates requiring mechanical ventilation are accustomed to witnessing very rapid changes in their vital signs and

Table 2-2. Blood Gas Scoring System for Assisted Ventilation*
Ambient Oxygen Failure → CPAP
CPAP Failure (CPAP 10 CM H_2O and 100% F_iO_2) → IPPV

	0	1	2	3
PaO_2	>60	50–60	<50**	<50
pH	>7.30	7.20–7.29	7.10–7.19	<7.10
$PaCO_2$	<50	50–60	61–70	>70

* A score of 3 or more indicates need for CPAP or IPPV.   ** May indicate need for CPAP or IPPV by itself, if cyanotic heart disease not present.

Adapted from: Goldsmith JP, Karotkin EH: Introduction to assisted ventilation. In: Assisted Ventilation of the Neonate, ed. Goldsmith JP, Karotkin EH. Philadelphia, WB Saunders, 1981.

Table 2-3. Classification System for
Ventilators

1. Cycle Mechanism
    a. Pressure
    b. Time
    c. Volume
2. Limit Mechanism (Preset)
    a. Pressure
    b. Volume

clinical condition. These rapid changes necessitate that those responsible intervene at the earliest possible moment when a problem with ventilation arises. A general understanding of how ventilators function will help the practitioners to anticipate and react quickly and appropriately to any deterioration in respiratory status.

Commercially available neonatal ventilators include both positive and negative pressure devices. Since negative pressure devices are used by a very small percentage of neonatal care facilities, this discussion will be limited to positive pressure ventilators which are categorized by how the positive pressure breath is cycled and limited. A basic classification scheme of ventilators is listed in Table 2-3. The majority of neonatal ventilators are cycled by pressure, time, or volume, and may be limited by pressure or volume. Cycling refers to the method by which inspiration is ended and exhalation is begun. The limiting parameter may be preset by the operator and determines either the maximum pressure or volume delivered to the infant. Table 2-4 lists the commonly used neonatal ventilators and their classifications.

Many features are common to currently used neonatal ventilators. Most have an air/oxygen mixing device that allows for gas delivery in concentrations from ambient to 100 percent oxygen. Neonatal ventilators also have a mechanism for the delivery of end expiratory pressure in conjunction with a mechanical rate (Positive End Expiratory Pressure, PEEP) or with the neonate breathing spontaneously (CPAP). Both pressure and volume ventilators have

Table 2-4. Neonatal Ventilators and Their Classifications

Pressure-Limited Ventilators	
Bear BP-200*	time-cycled, constant flow
Healthdyne 102, 105, 200	generator
Sechrist IV-100B	
Bio-Med MVP-10	pressure-cycled, constant flow
Bird Babybird	generator
Volume-Limited Ventilators	
Bear LS104-150*	time-cycled, constant flow
	generator
Emerson 3PV	time-cycled, non-constant flow
	generator
Siemens Servo 900B	time-cycled, constant or non-
	constant flow generator

* Previously known as Bourns Medical Systems.

a control by which the mechanical rate can be set. Most neonatal ventilators provide an IMV mode whereby the infant receives gas flow of the preset FiO_2 and end expiratory pressure interposed between mandatory mechanical breaths. This technique "allows precisely graded levels of support consistent with the degree of disease which is present"[12] and may force the infant to use his diaphragm, thus preventing disuse atrophy and aiding in weaning the infant from ventilatory support.[13]

The volume of gas generated with each breath is controlled differently with a pressure-limited ventilator than with a volume-limited ventilator. Pressure-limited ventilators allow a peak inspiratory pressure (PIP), an inspiratory time (T_i), and a flow rate to be preset. The volume of gas delivered (V_t) is determined primarily by the PIP and the infant's lung compliance. A decrease in compliance at a constant preset PIP results in a proportionate decrease in the delivered V_t. Conversely, an increase in the preset PIP at a constant lung compliance increases the delivered V_t. The ventilatory parameters of PIP, T_i and flow rate interact to affect the delivered V_t. Manipulating these parameters singularly or in combination with other ventilatory parameters may alter the delivered V_t but a discussion of how these alterations occur is beyond the scope of this chapter.

In comparison, a volume-limited ventilator allows the V_t and T_i to be preset or directly controlled. This results in the delivery of a constant V_t. The PIP resulting from the delivery of a set volume of gas in a set period of time is variable and is measured by a pressure manometer on the ventilator.

The inspiratory to expiratory ratio (I/E ratio) is determined by the setting of a desired rate and inspiratory time. This ventilatory parameter is a ratio of the time allotted for inspiration to occur compared to the time allotted for expiration. Many neonatal ventilators display this parameter as a result of the rate and inspiratory time settings. An increase in the I/E ratio results in an increase in the amount of time allotted for inspiration, thereby directly increasing the MAP.

Overview of Ventilatory Techniques

The advent of a more varied approach to neonatal mechanical ventilation has created the need to define these techniques more specifically and uniformly. This can be done fairly simply by using the ventilatory parameter of mechanical rate to delineate specific ventilatory techniques currently used. Table 2-5 shows this classification scheme as described by Fox and others. The first of these four classifications, slow rate ventilation, generally involves the use of a mechanical rate in the range of 20–40 breaths per minute. Rapid rate ventilation involves the use of a mechanical rate in the 60–80 breath per minute range. Both of these methods have been employed effectively in the ventilation of neonates with the primary diagnosis of RDS. Mechanical rates above 80 breaths per minute have been advocated for the treatment of PPHN. The use of these rates generally in the 100–150 breath per minute range has been termed hyperventilation since the primary objective is to lower the arterial partial pres-

Table 2-5. Classification of Ventilatory Techniques

Slow rate	20–40 BPM*
Rapid rate	60–80 BPM
Hyperventilation	100–150 BPM
High Frequency	300–1800 BPM

* BPM = Breaths per minute.

sure of carbon dioxide ($PaCO_2$). A detailed discussion of all three of these methods may be found in the section on Controversies in Neonatal Mechanical Ventilation.

The final classification category includes the use of rates in the range of 300–1800 breaths per minute. This technique is termed high frequency oscillatory ventilation and remains very much in the research stages of development, although there is much interest in its potential application (see Future Trends).

CONTROVERSIES IN METHODS OF VENTILATION

The techniques used in neonatal ventilatory support vary among neonatal centers as do the types of ventilators employed to provide this support. Hakanson describes the ideal ventilator as one that "will maintain constant ventilation despite changes in compliance and resistance."[13] Currently available mechanical ventilators all attempt to meet this goal but do so with limited success. Therefore, it remains incumbent upon caregivers to detect these changes in lung mechanics and to alter mechanical ventilation accordingly. This section will discuss controversies in approaches to ventilation for compliance disease (RDS) and the somewhat controversial technique of hyperventilation for the treatment of PPHN.

Pressure Versus Volume Ventilation

Neonatal ventilation deals mostly with an attempt to expand already collapsed pulmonary airways and alveoli associated with compliance disease. The pressure required to expand these areas of collapse is often extremely high. The advantages and disadvantages of pressure-oriented and volume-oriented ventilation for compliance disease as outlined by Fox and Hakanson in *Assisted Ventilation of the Neonate* are listed in Table 2-6.

Fox contends that while no definite studies demonstrate a physiologic advantage of either method, a pressure-limited ventilator may have an edge in coping with an almost pure compliance problem. Recent data suggest that PIP is implicated in the occurrence of pulmonary barotrauma and BPD.[15] Therefore, the ability to control and limit inspiratory pressure may be desirable and is simpler to achieve with a pressure-limited ventilator. A drawback of limiting the PIP with pressure-limited ventilation is the variability of the delivered V_t with changes in lung compliance. The V_t will decrease proportionally to a fall

Table 2-6. Advantages and Disadvantages of Pressure-Oriented and Volume Oriented Ventilation

Pressure-Oriented Ventilation

Advantages:
    1. Constant pressure delivered with each breath
    2. Safety: preset PIP
    3. Simpler design and operation
    4. Compact size and mobility
    5. Relatively inexpensive
Disadvantages:
    1. Variability of delivered V_t with changes in lung compliance

Volume-Oriented Ventilation

Advantages:
    1. Constant volume delivered with each breath
    2. Safety: preset V_t
    3. Less complicated mode of action
Disadvantages:
    1. Variability of delivered V_t to lungs of nonuniform compliance

in lung compliance and may result in serious hypoventilation if not recognized quickly. Recognition of compliance changes depends primarily on frequent blood gas analysis. However, the ability to measure TPP may make the detection of compliance changes easier and available on a more continuous basis.

The use of a volume-limited ventilator generates a constant tidal volume. Hakanson reports a distinct safety advantage with presetting the V_t as opposed to the PIP. Excess volume, not pressure, is thought to directly cause alveolar rupture so that controlling this parameter may offer an advantage. Yet the constant V_t generated by a volume-oriented ventilator may lead to preferential ventilation of the more compliant normal areas of the infant lung. Thus, areas of poor compliance and collapse remain atelectatic and under-ventilated. A neonate with a large portion of atelectatic lung volume develops a large intrapulmonary shunt which results in hypoxemia and eventually hypercarbia.

The delivered V_t, whether by mechanical or manual means, depends on two factors: (1) the mechanical properties of the lungs (such as compliance and resistance); and (2) the volume of air leaking around the endotracheal tube with each positive pressure breath. A change in either factor alters the volume of gas available to participate in gas exchange. As discussed previously, the neonate's compliance can change rapidly and dramatically. The second factor, the presence of an air leak around the endotracheal tube, confounds the task of delivering a constant V_t and is unpreventable and variable in the neonate. This is because the size and fragility of the neonatal trachea prohibit the use of cuffed endotracheal tubes for this age group. Therefore, delivery of a constant and measurable V_t is a difficult task at best and requires careful auscultatory assessment to help evaluate the significance of the volume loss.

The recognition of the need to control and closely monitor the pressures used in providing mechanical ventilatory support has led to the use of volume-limited ventilators as something other than true volume ventilators. Many practitioners preset a pressure limit, thereby making a volume-limited ventilator essentially pressure-limited. Likewise, some practitioners "convert" a pressure-limited ventilator into a volume-oriented machine by making the pressure limit artificially high and limiting ventilation in terms of maximum flow rate and inspiratory time. This technique may be useful when ventilating larger infants where lung compliance is relatively normal and tidal volume is more reasonably measured.

The controversy about the best method for facilitating the most effective gas exchange with the least amount of pulmonary damage will continue to evolve as practitioners pursue this goal.

Slow Rate Versus Rapid Rate Ventilation

Recently two distinct approaches to mechanical ventilation for compliance disease have evolved. The main contrasting feature is a difference in the range of ventilatory rates. Advocates of the slow rate method (20 to 30 breaths per minute) employ an inspiratory time of at least one second and moderate levels of PIP (less than 30 cm H_2O) and PEEP (less than 8 cm H_2O). Practitioners who employ the rapid rate technique (60 to 80 breaths per minute) utilize a shorter inspiratory time of approximately a half second with moderate levels of PIP and PEEP.

Reynolds, an advocate of slow rate ventilation, recommends the use of a prolonged inspiratory time in conjunction with a slow rate not greater than 30 breaths per minute to achieve effective neonatal mechanical ventilation.[16] He describes three methods to increase mean airway pressure in the face of an unacceptable PaO_2 whose effects may be additive. The most preferred method is to further prolong the T_i, for example, from an I/E ratio of 1:1 to 2:1. Reynolds advocates this method first since an increase in PIP may cause unacceptable pulmonary damage or barotrauma. If the PaO_2 continues to be low, Reynolds employs a small increase in PEEP along with a small increase in PIP and a further increase in I/E ratio. He then increases these parameters in concert if the PaO_2 remains refractory. He feels that significant improvements in PaO_2 are possible with this approach and that this improvement may be maintained during the weaning process.

Reynolds has reported trials of rapid rate ventilation for compliance disease but has found that this method did not adequately oxygenate neonates with severe hyaline membrane disease.[17] Advocates of the rapid rate method are quick to point out, however, that these trials were carried out before the use of PEEP. In 1977, Sjostrand advocated the use of rapid rates as a method to minimize the effects of positive pressure ventilation on cardiovascular function, seen as an elevation of mean intrathoracic pressure and decreased venous return resulting in decreased cardiac output.[18]

Hiecher, Kasting, and Harrod have reported a prospective clinical comparison of the two methods of neonatal ventilation.[19] From this study of 102 infants, the authors have shown no difference in mortality, time requiring ventilation, or the incidence of patent ductus arteriosis or chronic lung disease.

They did show a difference in two categories that may be potentially significant. Mean starting and highest PIP were significantly lower for the group that was ventilated using the rapid rate technique. In addition, there was a difference in the number of infants who developed pneumothoraces, with a 14 percent occurrence in the rapid group and a 35 percent occurrence in the slow rate group. These two differences may prove significant for those who are responsible for neonatal ventilation but further documentation of these findings is essential.

Mechanical rates in excess of 80 breaths per minute have no place in the current practice of mechanical ventilation for compliance disease. Above this rate, poorly compliant areas of the neonatal lung cannot empty in the short time allotted for exhalation. Air trapping and profound hypercapnia occur and the potential for alveolar rupture results. Rates above 80 are best utilized in hyperventilation where pulmonary hypertension is the primary diagnosis.

Hyperventilation Therapy for PPHN

The use of the technique of hyperventilation for the treatment of persistent pulmonary hypertension of the neonate (PPHN) has gained acceptance in many neonatal intensive care units. PPHN is characterized by an increase in pulmonary artery pressure above systemic artery pressure, causing restricted pulmonary blood flow or significant right-to-left intracardiac shunting of unsaturated blood through the foramen ovale and/or the ductus arteriosus. This condition can result in profound hypoxemia that is unresponsive to increases in levels of F_iO_2 or PEEP. Factors that increase pulmonary vascular resistance by vasoconstriction are bradykinin, hypoxemia, acidosis and hypercarbia. The use of ventilator rates between 100-150 breaths per minute have been shown to effectively control pulmonary artery pressure by decreasing the $PaCO_2$ to as low as 20 torr.[6] This technique reduces pulmonary vascular resistance and thus reverses the right-to-left shunt more consistently than any of the pulmonary vasodilators currently available.[20] Furthermore, hyperventilation therapy does not have the potentially serious side effects associated with some of the vasodilators—one of which is the tendency to drop systemic arterial pressure below optimal levels.

In conjunction with these ventilatory rates, Peckham and Fox have demonstrated the need for peak inspiratory pressures as high as 40-60 cm H_2O to lower the $PaCO_2$ to levels sufficient to reduce pulmonary artery pressures below systemic arterial pressures. This reduction is the key in reversing the profound hypoxemia that characterizes this disease.

The identification of a "critical level of $PaCO_2$" is a second key point in the treatment of PPHN described by Peckham and Fox. They report that this level is identifiable on an individual basis by finding the $PaCO_2$ above which the PaO_2 begins to fall precipitously. This critical level needs to be identified early in the disease process and maintained throughout the acute state of PPHN by whatever rate and PIP are necessary.

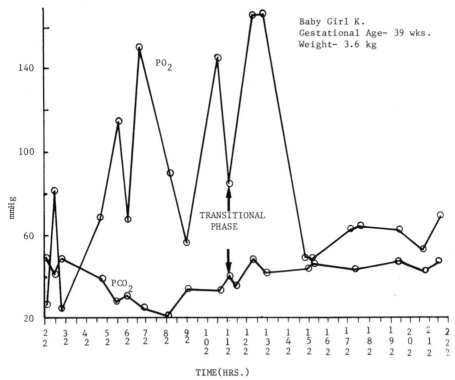

Fig. 2-5. Demonstration of PO_2 lability before transitional phase, and decreased PCO_2 responsiveness after transitional phase in PPHN. F_iO_2 1.0 until 142 hours, then .7. At transitional phase, PIP decreased from 50–35 cmH_2O and RR from 150-30 BPM.

The advent of neonatal ventilators with the ability to ventilate at rates to 150 breaths per minute has allowed for the ventilation of neonates mechanically rather than manually as was often necessary in the past. The use of more rapid rates may allow the clinician to achieve the desired $PaCO_2$ at lower peak pressures than might be necessary at slower rates and reduce the risk of barotrauma associated with higher peak pressures.

Since 1978 when the study describing the treatment of PPHN by hyperventilation was published, research has revealed further information on weaning the neonate from hyperventilation. Sosulski and Fox have described that during the course of PPHN treated by hyperventilation, a "transitional phase" usually occurs two or three days after the initiation of hyperventilation (Figure 2-5).[21] The hypoxemia that heretofore was the result of extrapulmonary shunting now becomes secondary to pulmonary parenchymal disease. Once this transitional phase occurs, the $PaCO_2$ may rise above the critical level without a concomitant fall in the PaO_2. The chances of barotrauma are highest at this point and the patient must be weaned carefully but quickly to avoid its occurrence. Further research is necessary to more clearly identify this transitional phase as it occurs during the course of PPHN.

Critics of this method for the treatment of PPHN cite the lack of follow-up data presently available for neonates treated using hyperventilation.[22] The possible neurologic sequelae of the prolonged alkalemic state seen with hyperventilation has been questioned. The cause for concern is that hypocarbia decreases cerebral blood flow and potentiates the possibility of cerebral hypoxia. In a recent study of 12 infants who had been treated with hyperventilation therapy with $PaCO_2$ levels less than 30 torr for a mean of 15 hours and peak inflating pressures greater than 30 cm H_2O for a mean of 102 hours, a low incidence of severe neurodevelopmental problems resulting from the disease or its therapy was found.[23]

ADJUNCTIVE NON-INVASIVE MONITORING FOR MECHANICAL VENTILATION

Along with the development and refinement of neonatal mechanical ventilators, monitoring equipment (both invasive and more recently non-invasive) has been developed to aid the bedside clinician by providing data that was previously unavailable. Sophisticated devices such as transcutaneous gas analyzers, end tidal CO_2 analyzers and airway pressure monitors have come into clinical use in many neonatal intensive care units. These devices have allowed the neonatal practitioner to reliably and continuously monitor the effectiveness of the ventilation being provided.

Transcutaneous Monitoring Devices

A decade has passed since the first data on the application of a miniaturized, heated Clark electrode for the measurement of oxygen tension at the skin surface appeared in the literature. This data was published simultaneously by two groups, Huch et al[24] and Eberhard et al.[25] Since that time, the transcutaneous oxygen electrode has been widely accepted in many neonatal intensive units.

Many clinicians have assumed that transcutaneous oxygen partial pressures ($PtcO_2$ or $TcPO_2$) and PaO_2 are equal to each other. This assumption has been supported by many early studies revealing a high correlation co-efficient between the two values. In the stable neonate, $P_{tc}O_2$ monitoring has been shown to approximate PaO_2 very closely. However, in the critically ill neonate, $P_{tc}O_2$ monitoring has often been found unreliable in a situation where continuous monitoring of this nature could be extremely helpful.[26]

Clinicians who have continued to use this non-invasive device on a regular basis have found that it is additionally useful in tracking the PaO_2 consistently over a wide range of infants over an extended period of time. Studies have shown that divergence of the $PtcO_2$ and the PaO_2 may indicate some degree of circulatory impairment. The amount of divergence may give the clinician valuable information about the severity of circulatory impairment. The measurement of $PtcO_2$ depends on peripheral blood flow to the site of the electrode which warms the skin and enhances flow. Thus, a drop in $PtcO_2$ may represent significant vasoconstriction.

Establishment and documentation of a baseline correlation between $PtcO_2$ and PaO_2 is essential prior to monitoring a neonate continuously through a critical, life-threatening episode that results in a drop in the measured $PtcO_2$. Then, if an arterial blood gas indicates a corresponding fall in the PaO_2, the neonate has respiratory impairment. If the PaO_2 remains essentially unchanged, the neonate has suffered some degree of circulatory impairment.[26] By using this technique, the clinician can determine the appropriate alterations in the treatment regimen that are necessary.

The nurse can utilize $PtcO_2$ monitoring in a variety of circumstances to aid in the assessment of the neonate's status. For example, the $PtcO_2$ may drop precipitously in response to cold stress-related vasoconstriction. The $PtcO_2$ electrode may also be used to evaluate the effect of the many nursing interventions that are necessary for the infant undergoing mechanical ventilation. Such common interventions as broncho-pulmonary segmental drainage, endotracheal suctioning, nasogastric feedings, and weighing an infant in addition to other factors such as noise levels in the unit can have a direct effect on the PaO_2 of a neonate. The use of transcutaneous oxygen monitoring can reveal how well the infant is tolerating these procedures and alert practitioners to the need for intervention such as identifying and reducing stressful situations when possible. It can also be used to evaluate the effects of planned care and soothing actions by the staff and family.

Another direct application of $PtcO_2$ monitoring concerns the diagnostic evaluation of the presence of shunting in a neonate suspected of having PPHN. By placing two $PtcO_2$ electrodes on the infant, one preductally (upper right trunk) and one postductally (left hemithorax or below nipple line), the presence and degree of right-to-left shunting occurring at the level of the ductus arteriosis can be determined. This can eliminate the necessity of determining the actual PaO_2 at these two levels by invasive and, therefore, more difficult and risky techniques.

More recently, a second transcutaneous measuring device has been developed that utilizes the Stowe-Severinghaus carbon dioxide electrode in a miniaturized form. This electrode measures transcutaneous partial pressures of carbon dioxide ($PtcCO_2$ or $TcpCO_2$) and once again has been quickly scrutinized as to its ability to equal the $PaCO_2$. Numerous evaluations have found that $PtcCO_2$ values were consistently higher than $PaCO_2$. This is because the transcutaneous CO_2 electrode actually measures tissue PCO_2 which is expected to be higher than arterial PO_2. A gradient between concentrations of CO_2 in the tissue and blood must exist so that CO_2 produced locally will be removed. Barring circulatory changes similar to those described earlier for $PtcO_2$, the difference between $PtcCO_2$ and $PaCO_2$ remains constant over time in the same patient.[27] This point emphasizes the importance of establishing a baseline correlation between transcutaneous and arterial values early in the course of $PtcO_2$ monitoring.

The application of $PtcCO_2$ monitoring in the neonate being mechanically ventilated has been described by Hansen and Tooley.[28] They have found that the "skin surface PCO_2 electrode has been helpful in the management of infants being mechanically ventilated, allowing for better control of PCO_2 than was possible when $PaCO_2$ was being intermittently measured." As with the $PtcO_2$ monitor, the effect of routine procedures performed frequently on the PCO_2 can be evaluated on a continuous basis. In addition, episodes of wide variations in PCO_2 not seen with intermittent measurement of the $PaCO_2$ can be recorded and documented.

A key point that applies to both PO_2 and PCO_2 determinations by transcutaneous techniques involves the use of these devices in place of arterial blood gas sampling. As was emphasized earlier, a determination of the correlation with arterial values is essential to the proper use of these devices. Without this initial comparison and subsequent comparisons with significant changes in the clinical condition of the neonate, the reliability of the data obtained is questionable.

End-Tidal Carbon Dioxide Monitoring

End-tidal CO_2 monitoring has been in use in adult and pediatric intensive care settings for the past few years. Its value in providing information leading to an estimate of $PaCO_2$ is dependent upon the ability to obtain a true alveolar air sample. The PCO_2 of alveolar gas is equivalent to $PaCO_2$ in the absence of pulmonary disease. If a true alveolar sample is obtained, the derived PCO_2 value may then be compared with the $PaCO_2$ value obtained from an arterial blood sample. In a manner similar to that of transcutaneous monitoring, a correlation between end-tidal CO_2 and $PaCO_2$ is established. Barring significant changes in pulmonary status, the end-tidal CO_2 may then be used to "trend" the $PaCO_2$ continuously and non-invasively.

The application of this monitoring device to neonatal pulmonary care has been impeded by two factors. First, the connections to the neonatal airway are usually so large that they represent a significant portion of the neonate's V_t. This increase in total deadspace may result in rebreathing of the volume in the adapter leading to an artificially high end-tidal CO_2 reading. The second limitation is the ability of the monitor to sample at the frequency many neonates breathe. With too rapid a respiratory rate, the monitor will yield an inaccurate result on the low side.

End-tidal CO_2 has yet to make a significant impact on neonatal pulmonary care. The limitations of the device when applied to neonates restricts its widespread application as a reliable estimate of $PaCO_2$.

Airway Pressure Monitoring

Another device that has come into use as a monitoring adjunct for the infant being mechanically ventilated is one that determines various airway pressure parameters and displays them on a continuous basis. Such a device is shown in Figure 2-6. Airway pressure monitors have the ability to measure mean airway pressure, a parameter that has become very significant in recent years primarily because of its effect on increasing the PaO_2. Many alterations in ventilatory parameters are currently being expressed in terms of their effect on MAP.

Reynolds described various techniques for increasing MAP in reporting his methods of neonatal mechanical ventilation.[16] Others have also reported the importance of this variable in determining oxygenation. Unfortunately, an absolute value for MAP that will insure good oxygenation has not been reported in the literature. It has been shown that an increase in MAP improves oxygenation up to a point and that many variables affect MAP (see Table 2-7). The effect of alterations in PIP, PEEP, T_i, and I/E ratio on MAP and oxygenation was the subject of a recently published study.[29] The investigators found that increases in PEEP lead to the greatest change in PaO_2 per change in MAP ($\Delta PaO_2/\Delta MAP$), followed by increases in PIP and I/E ratio using a pressure-limited ventilator.

Increasing MAP to improve oxygenation is not without potential detriment to the neonate. In a recent study of nine neonates with the diagnosis of respiratory distress syndrome, it was shown that a direct relationship exists between the MAP necessary to provide adequate oxygenation and the severity of the lung pathology.[30] In addition, the investigators found that complications should be anticipated when a MAP of greater than 12 cmH$_2$O is required.

Transpulmonary pressure (TPP), another airway pressure variable which has had limited application in the neonatal intensive care unit, is a variable determined by the use of a catheter with an external inflatable balloon that is placed in the distal third of the esophagus. This catheter is attached to a transducer that measures the pressure existing in this portion of the esophagus during the ventilatory cycle.

As mentioned earlier, TPP is an expression of the difference between the delivered pressure and that measured in the esophagus. When transpulmonary pressure increases, less pressure is being transmitted to the pleural space, hence lung compliance is worsening. When TPP decreases, more of the delivered pressure is being transmitted and lung compliance is improving. The significance of knowing when changes in lung compliance are occurring is that the clinician may then make the appropriate changes in ventilation to reduce the risk of barotrauma or avoid a worsening in the pulmonary status of the neonate. TPP may also have an additional application in the identification of

Table 2-7. Factors That Affect MAP

Distending Pressure

    PEEP, CPAP, PIP

Duration of Positive Pressure

    Inspiratory Time
    I/E Ratio

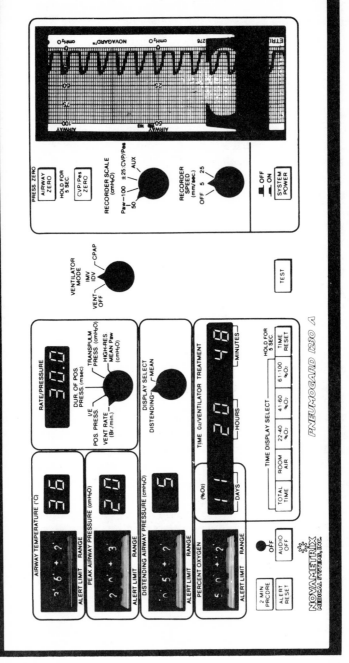

Fig. 2-6. Novametrix Pneumogard 1230A Ventilation Monitor (courtesy of Novametrix Medical Systems, Inc. Wallingford, Ct.)

the transitional phase occurring during the treatment of PPHN (see Controversies Section).

FUTURE TRENDS IN NEONATAL MECHANICAL VENTILATION

High Frequency Oscillatory Ventilation

A new ventilatory technique has received much attention in the literature yet remains in the research stages. This technique employs the use of rates generally in the 300–1800 breath per minute range (5–30 Hz, or Cycles Per Second) and has been termed high frequency oscillatory ventilation.

High frequency oscillatory ventilation has been successfully accomplished in animal studies by the use of a piston pump. This pump is capable of generating high frequency, small-volume, sinusoidal oscillations at the patient airway. Bohn et al have used this method in the ventilation of paralyzed, anesthetized dogs and found that excellent gas exchange could be achieved using volumes much smaller than that of the deadspace.[31] The investigators further determined that the optimal frequency for CO_2 elimination was 15 Hz using volumes of 1.0 ml/kg and generating peak inspiratory pressures of 4–8 cmH$_2$O. These ventilatory parameters clearly suggest that gas exchange using high frequency oscillatory ventilation must be occurring by a different method than that achieved with conventional ventilation.

Gas transport through the conducting airways and down to the level of the terminal bronchioles and alveoli is generally thought to occur by bulk flow. Diffusion is thought to play a major role in gas transport only when the gas reaches this level. The use of high frequency oscillation as a means of mechanical ventilation as described by Bohn and others is thought to conduct gas to the alveoli by some form of facilitated diffusion rather than by bulk flow. The basis for this theory is that bulk flow cannot occur since the tidal volumes used are up to four times less than the volume of the dead space.

The potential applications of this method to neonatal mechanical ventilation are very significant. With conventional ventilation, volumes of gas sufficient to insure adequate gas exchange must be delivered with fairly high pressures to a lung of nonuniform compliance. This can lead to overdistension of the more compliant areas with the resultant risk of significant pulmonary barotrauma.[11] If gas exchange can be accomplished in the neonate utilizing high frequency oscillations that deliver small tidal volumes with minimal peak airway pressures, the occurrence of pulmonary barotrauma may be drastically reduced.

Data recently published on a trial of high frequency oscillation in eight neonates with severe respiratory distress syndrome supports this conclusion.[32] In this study, low-volume, high-frequency oscillations were delivered through standard endotracheal tubes. The frequencies utilized varied between 8 and 20 Hz, with mean airway pressures between 9 and 20 cmH$_2$O. The investigators demonstrated improvement in oxygenation with high frequency oscillation such that the FiO_2 was reduced from 0.66 ± 0.15 to 0.41 ± 0.11 to provide similar PaO_2s. These improvements in oxygenation correlated directly with increases in MAP. The increases seen in MAP were not associated with an increased risk of barotrauma since these increases were achieved with a markedly smaller tidal volume and PIP.

The data supplied in this preliminary report on the application of high frequency oscillation to the treatment of neonatal pulmonary disease is most encouraging. However, many questions are unanswered concerning the necessity and the method for proper humidification of gas delivered to the patient airway in this manner, among others.

The implications of this new ventilatory technique for the critical care nurse are many. In addition to gaining familiarity with a completely different means for providing ventilation, the nurse will need to refine and possibly alter current respiratory assessment skills to care for the neonate ventilated in this manner. The delivery of low-volume, high frequency oscillations will present a sharp contrast to the visible and measureable chest wall movements and auscultative findings that occur with conventional ventilation. Pulmonary care techniques such as endotracheal suctioning may need to be changed to allow for the continued delivery of oscillatory ventilation. Additionally, these skills will involve the reliance upon sophisticated monitoring adjuncts requiring personnel trained to monitor their use and interpret the data. This will likely increase the interdependence of health care personnel responsible for neonatal pulmonary care.

Surfactant: Prenatal and Postnatal Considerations

Two areas that seem promising are the acceleration of fetal lung maturation and the therapeutic use of surfactant in HMD. Investigations are underway to develop and refine methods to accomplish these goals. Currently, therapy to enhance lung maturation involves administration of adrenal corticosteroids to the mother. This method has a moderate rate of success. Numerous factors are associated with its effectiveness. Moreover, the long term effects on the infant are unkown at this time.

The use of topical surfactant therapy in premature neonates with RDS has received worldwide attention. Initial experimental and clinical trials with an aerosol of the principal component of pulmonary surfactant proved uniformly ineffective. Further studies indicated that delivery of "natural" surfactant to the lung of fetal animals before the onset of breathing, seemed to compensate for a deficiency of alveolar surfactant. However, side effects and variable specific surface activity prevent its use in man. Lyophilized artificial surfactant has been developed and its endotracheal instillation in preterm infants with HMD has been demonstrated to improve pulmonary function and hasten recovery.[33] A breakthrough in these areas is hoped to significantly alter the severity and management of neonatal pulmonary disease and its associated mortality and morbidity.

SUMMARY

The technologic and therapeutic advances that have occurred over the past two decades in the field of neonatology suggest a bright and eventful future. How the practitioners of the future will master the new knowledge, devices, and techniques that are certain to develop will determine their roles.

The burden of providing the education to assume these future roles will continue to fall on the individual. Currently, programs offered nationwide emphasize this self-reliance approach to education. Many convey information from a variety of disciplines involved in a particular care specialty. Practitioners may thus gain a strong appreciation for many aspects that affect patient care that are not their direct responsibility.

This collaborative approach to continuing education also applies to direct patient care. Nursing and respiratory therapy staffs will assume responsibility for more of the technical skills and refined clinical assessments necessary to intervene promptly in critically ill neonates. These professionals are the closest to the infant and the most constantly involved persons. Therefore, they will implement these techniques and skills and be the most attuned to individual infant responses.

REFERENCES

1. Donald I, Lord J: Augmented respiration: studies in atelectasis neonatorum. Lancet 1:9, 1953
2. Gregory GA, Ketterman JA, Phibbs RH, et al: Treatment of the idiopathic respiratory distress syndrome with continuous positive airway pressure. N Engl J Med 284:1333, 1971
3. Chernick V, Vidyassagar D: Continuous chest wall pressure in hyaline membrane disease: One year experience. Pediatrics 49:753, 1972
4. Gerard P, Fox WW, Outerbridge EW, et al: Early versus late introduction of continuous negative pressure in the management of idiopathic respiratory distress syndrome. J Pediatr 87:591, 1979
5. Downs JB, Klein LF, Desautels D, et al: Intermittent mandatory ventilation: A new approach to weaning patients from mechanical ventilation. Chest 64:331, 1973
6. Peckham GJ, Fox WW: Physiological factors affecting pulmonary artery pressure in infants with persistent pulmonary hypertension. J Pediatr 93:1005, 1978
7. Emery JL, Mitwal A: The number of alveoli in the terminal respiratory unit in man during late intrauterine life and childhood. Arch Dis Child 35:544, 1960
8. Harris TR: Physiological principles. In: Assisted Ventilation of the Neonate, ed. Goldsmith JP, Karotkin EH. Philadelphia, W.B. Saunders, 1981
9. Williams SM: The pulmonary system. In: The Core Curriculum for Critical Care Nurses, 2ed, eds Borg N et al. The American Association of Critical-Care Nurses. Philadelphia, W.B. Saunders 1981

10. Reynolds O: Ventilatory therapy. In: Neonatal Pulmonary Care, ed. Thibeault DW, Gregory GA. Menlo Park, Addision-Wesley, 1979
11. Goldsmith JP, Karotkin EH: Introduction to assisted ventilation. In: Assisted Ventilation of the Neonate, ed. Goldsmith JP, Karotkin EH. Philadelphia, W.B. Saunders, 1981
12. Polgar GE: Mechanical properties of lung and chest wall. In: Neonatal Pulmonary Care, ed. Thibeault DW, Gregory GA. Menlo Park, Addison-Wesley, 1979
13. Kirby RR: Design of mechanical ventilators. In: Neonatal Pulmonary Care, ed. Thibeault DW, Gregory GA. Menlo Park, Addison-Wesley, 1979
14. Hakanson DO: Positive pressure ventilation: Volume-cycled ventilators. In: Assisted Ventilation of the Neonate, ed. Goldsmith JP, Karotkin EH. Philadelphia, W.B. Saunders, 1981
15. Reynolds EOR, Taghizadeh A: Improved prognosis of infants mechanically ventilated for hyaline membrane disease. Arch Dis Child 49:505, 1974
16. Reynolds EOR: Pressure waveform and ventilator settings for mechanical ventilation in severe hyaline membrane disease. Bourns Educational Series ES1
17. Reynolds EOR: Effect of alterations in mechanical ventilator settings on pulmonary gas exchange in hyaline membrane disease. Arch Dis Child 46:152, 1971
18. Sjostrand U: Review of the physiological rationale for and development of high-frequency positive-pressure ventilation-HPPV. Acta Anesthesiol Scad Suppl 64:7, 1977
19. Heicher DA, Kastings DS, Harrod Jr: Prospective clinical comparison of two methods for mechanical ventilation of neonates: Rapid rate and short inspiratory time versus slow rate and long inspiratory time. J Pediatr 98:957, 1981
20. Drummond WH, Gregory GA, Heymann MA, et al: The independent effects of hyperventilation, tolazoline, and dopamine on infants with persistent pulmonary hypertension. J Pediatr 98:603, 1971
21. Fox WW: Mechanical ventilation in the management of persistent pulmonary hypertension. 83rd Ross Conference on Pediatric Research, June, 1980
22. King TD: Cardiovascular aspects. In: Assisted Ventilation of the Neonate, ed. Goldsmith JP, Karotkin EH. Philadelphia, W.B. Saunders, 1981
23. Bernbaum J, Russel P, Gewitz M, Fox WW, Peckham GJ: Neurodevelopmental and cardiorespiratory follow up of infants with persistent hypertension of the newborn. Ped Res 15:651, 1981
24. Huch A, Huch R, Lucey JF: Continuous transcutaneous blood gas monitoring. First International Symposium. Birth Defects: Original Article Series 15:1, 1979
25. Eberhard P, Mindt W, Kreuzer F: Cutaneous oxygen monitoring in the newborn. Pediatrician 5:335, 1976
26. Shoemaker WC, Vidyasagar D: Physiological and clinical significance of $PtcO_2$ and $PtcCO_2$ measurements. Crit Care Med 9:689, 1981
27. Cabal L, Hodgman J, Siassi B, et al: Factors affecting heated transcutaneous PO_2 and unheated transcutaneous PCO_2 in preterm infants. Crit Care Med 9:298, 1981
28. Hansen TN, Tooley WH: Skin surface carbon dioxide tension in sick infants. Pediatrics 64:942, 1979
29. Stewart AR, Finer NN, Peters KL: Effects of alterations of inspiratory and expiratory pressures and inspiratory/expiratory ratios on mean airway pressure, blood gases, and intracranial pressure. Pediatrics 67:474, 1981
30. Ciszek TA, Modanlou HD, Owings D, et al: Mean airway pressure-significance during mechanical ventilation in neonates. J Pediatr 99:121, 1981

31. Bohn DJ, Miyasaka K, Marchak BE, et al: Ventilation by high-frequency oscil-lation. J Appl Physiol 48:210, 1980
32. Marchak BE, Thompson WK, Duffy P, et al: Treatment of RDS by high-frequency oscillatory ventilation: A preliminary report. J Pediatr 99:287, 1981
33. Fujiwara T, Chida S, Watabe Y, et al: Artificial surfactant therapy in hyaline membrane disease. Lancet 1(8159):55, 1980

3 Current Considerations for Patent Ductus Arteriosus in the Critically Ill Newborn

Kit Stahler-Miller
Michael H. Gewitz

While much current medical research is focused on evaluating and manipulating the patent ductus arteriosus (PDA) in early infancy, its presence as a complication of prematurity has been recognized for many years. The first association of respiratory distress and patency of the ductus in premature infants was made by Bernard over 20 years ago.[1] Since then, advances in the treatment of both premature and fullterm newborns with congenital heart disease have made it increasingly important for medical personnel dealing with these critically ill infants to understand the physiologic implications and management considerations involving the ductus arteriosus. This chapter will review some of the recent information accumulated about the ductus and explain the relevance of this research to nursing and medical management decisions in the critical care nursery.

INCIDENCE

Several recent studies have reported that the incidence of PDA varies widely depending on gestational age, birth weight, and management details

Table 3-1. Incidence Figures for PDA in Premature Infants

Study	Weight (g)	% Patients with PDA
Kitterman (1972)	1750	15%
Neal (1975)	1500–2000	27%
	>2000	15%
Siassi (1976)	2000	36%
Stevenson (1977)	<2000	50%
Nadas (1981)	≤1750	20%

such as ventilatory status and fluid balance.[2–6] Table 3-1 reviews the incidence of PDA in several of these studies of preterm infants. Generally, an inverse relationship exists between gestational age and frequency of PDA; that is, the presence of a PDA is more likely in premature than in fullterm infants. Also a direct relationship exists between the severity of respiratory distress syndrome, which is synonymous with hyaline membrane disease, and the presence of PDA. Although these studies noted a 70–80% incidence in infants under 28–30 weeks gestational age, overall, 32% of infants under 36 weeks of age have evidence of a hemodynamically significant PDA (see section on diagnosis, below).

ROLE OF THE DUCTUS IN FETAL AND TRANSITIONAL CIRCULATION

The fetal ductus arteriosus (DA) is a large-caliber vessel that connects the pulmonary artery and the aorta and seems to have two functions. First, it serves as a bypass of the lungs; in utero these organs are fluid-filled and non-aerated, have a high pulmonary vascular resistance (PVR), and receive a relatively small percentage of cardiac output. A second—and more speculative—role of the DA is that of a volume "unloader" for the left ventricle. Studies have shown that the fetal heart may have limited ability to respond to increased pressure and volume loads as compared with the adult heart. Since the ductus diverts blood ejected by the right ventricle directly to the descending aorta, it thus limits volume loading of the left ventricle.[7]

Intrauterine factors that help to maintain ductal patency are relative hypoxemia plus the vasodilating action of prostaglandins (PGs), specifically PGI_2. The relationship of the prostaglandin pathway to ductal patency is a relatively recent discovery and still requires further elucidation. Previously it was believed that the ductus was kept open passively by transluminal pressure.

As gestation ends and delivery begins, a new phase of physiologic considerations that accompany the infant's change from intrauterine to extrauterine life affect ductal patency. At birth, the effect of inspired oxygen on the pulmonary and systemic circuits becomes significant. In general, increased oxygen saturation tends to increase systemic vascular resistance (SVR) via direct effects on peripheral vascular smooth muscle and tends to decrease pulmonary vascular resistance (PVR) by dilating the pulmonary vascular bed. Two other factors that are involved in the systemic vascular changes accompanying birth are the severance of the umbilical cord and the constricting effect of oxygen locally on the umbilical artery and ductal wall. Other mechanisms that bring about the pulmonary vascular changes are the operation of the lungs as a respiratory organ, and the consequent clearance of lung water, expansion of alveoli, and increase in the cross-sectional area of the pulmonary vascular bed. These factors initially help to reverse the flow of blood through the ductus and ultimately favor its closure.

CLOSURE MECHANISM

It has recently been postulated that the ductus arteriosus undergoes staged closure.[8] The early, or functional phase, usually occurs within the first 24 hrs of life in the term infant. Constriction is thought to be initiated by oxygen-related contraction of the smooth muscle in the wall of the ductus, with the pulmonary end closing first. Prostaglandin metabolism and perhaps other vasoactive agents also play a role in this process.[9,10] The late, or anatomic, phase usually occurs within a few days. Endothelial tissue deteriorates and granulation tissue proliferates to fill the ductus lumen, which then becomes the ligamentum arteriosus and is present throughout life.

Closure in preterm infants probably occurs by the same mechanisms but usually on a different timetable, generally happening when these infants reach the postnatal age and weight that corresponds to term gestational age and appropriate weight; however, immediate closure after birth in very immature infants may also occur. In these infants, however, the ductus may reopen after the contraction phase. Gittenberger-de Groot has identified four histologic maturation stages of ductal closure in preterm infants, implying that the closure mechanism is complex and is not complete until significant changes occur in cellular architecture. This information has significant bearing for medical manipulation of the ductus—such as with indomethacin—in the premature infant.[11] If such agents are administered soon after birth to infants in the early stages of ductal closure, complete anatomic closure may not result.

Delayed closure of the ductus in the fullterm newborn can occur in several conditions, which include certain forms of congenital heart diseases and the rubella syndrome, or can be an isolated event. This last type of persistent ductus, termed "pathologic PDA", appears to result from an underlying structural abnormality of the ductus itself and is unlikely to respond to chemical stimulation. It is distinct from persistent patency of the ductus in the preterm infant, which is thought to be characterized by an immature or poorly developed closure mechanism (see below) and is termed "PDA of immaturity". Chemical and mechanical closure of the ductus arteriosus will be discussed below.

THE PRETERM INFANT WITH RESPIRATORY
DISTRESS SYNDROME

The exact pathogenesis of persistent PDA in the premature infant is unknown, but several factors may be contributory. These include (1) decreased ductal responsiveness to oxygen, thought to be associated with immature enzyme systems; (2) low arterial oxygen tension (PaO_2) values, such as those often seen in premature infants with lung disease or in high-altitude settings; (3) an insufficient amount of muscle for adequate closure; and (4) an immature constriction response. Other causes may exist.

Several factors influence the clinical expression of PDA in the preterm infant with respiratory distress syndrome (RDS). Basically, the direction and magnitude of flow of the ductus (and perhaps its closure) depend on the size of the PDA and the relationship of pulmonary to systemic vascular resistance. Research involving the lamb fetus has demonstrated a relative underdevelopment of pulmonary arteriolar smooth muscle until late gestation. Thus, in the premature infant, PVR may be reduced and left-to-right shunting through the ductus could occur at an early postnatal age.[12] However, with RDS, operation of this shunt is variable because supervening hypoxia, hypercarbia, and acidosis may result in pulmonary vasoconstriction. Additional factors that may increase PVR are atelectasis (ATL) and positive-pressure ventilation. Moreover, mechanical ventilation may cause dissection of air outside the alveolus (pulmonary interstitial emphysema, PIE), which can mechanically obstruct pulmonary vessels by compression.

In summary, the clinical manifestations of PDA are most dependent on the instantaneous relationship between the pulmonary and systemic vascular beds. If PVR is high secondary to severe RDS, the shunt will be right-to-left. As PVR decreases, the shunt may be temporarily balanced. The infant may not exhibit clinical findings of PDA in either of these situations. In contrast, if PVR is low, a left-to-right shunt may be present even in the first few days of life. As mentioned, these factors are very dynamic and can fluctuate from moment to moment. A proposed feedback system involves the following: decreasing PVR allows an increase in pulmonary blood flow; this expanded flow results in increasing pulmonary vascular pressure and the amount of lung water, a result that increases the work of breathing. The infant tires and develops carbon dioxide retention and an oxygen deficit. Hypercarbia and hypoxemia then cause PVR to rise, and the flow of blood from the aorta to the lungs decreases.

DIAGNOSIS

Symptomatic PDA in the sick preterm infant is usually not difficult to diagnose. Many infants with hyaline membrane disease (HMD) who are below 32 weeks gestation and whose weight is appropriate for gestational age (AGA) develop evidence of PDA when the initial respiratory distress abates. The presenting signs of PDA can be respiratory. Just as the infant recovers from RDS, he suddenly worsens and develops the respiratory signs and symptoms of pulmonary edema, which may be strikingly similar to those that occur with RDS, including tachypnea, expiratory grunting, intercostal retractions, and difficulty with gas exchange. Fine, crackling râles, best heard with deep breaths, are usually a late finding and indicate significant pulmonary edema.

Murmurs, in this case reflective of turbulent blood flow through the ductus, can also develop. Two principle types of murmurs are associated with PDA. Classically, the continuous ("to and fro," or "machinery") murmur in the upper left precordium is the hallmark of the ductus. The quality of this murmur is usually harsh, and it is heard throughout systole and through the second heart sound into diastole. The murmur is usually associated with a large PDA and represents the existence of significant flow throughout the cardiac cycle. In the preterm infant a PDA may also be represented by a systolic ejection murmur (SEM) alone without the diastolic component. This murmur is also usually heard in the upper left precordium but is usually of higher pitch and has a blowing quality; it is associated with a small or moderate sized PDA in which there is negligible diastolic flow.

Third and fourth heart sounds (S_3 and S_4) may be heard. A third sound (also called an S_3 gallop, a ventricular gallop, or a protodiastolic gallop) is the result of decreased ventricular compliance. A fourth sound (also called an S_4 gallop, an atrial gallop, or a presystolic gallop) reflects atrial contraction in the presence of a poorly compliant ventricle. An S_4 is usually very difficult to hear in a premature infant because of the rapid heart rate. Heart sounds and the intensity or quality of the murmur do not always reflect either the amount of shunting or the degree to which the PDA causes respiratory insufficiency.

Usually, infants with significant PDA have wide pulse pressures ("runoff") and may have resultant bounding peripheral pulses. The larger the left-to-right shunt, the more this becomes apparent. The mean diastolic pressure may become very low and jeopardize the coronary artery blood supply, which may result in myocardial ischemia. Additional findings may include tachycardia, which is a compensatory mechanism enabling increased cardiac output in the presence of volume overload from the left-to-right shunt, and hepatomegaly, which may reflect increased systemic venous pressures. This latter sign may be less reliable in the premature infant. Peripheral edema, which frequently accompanies congestive heart failure (CHF) in older children, is less often seen in premature infants unless associated with excessive administration of intravascular fluids or with hypoalbuminemia.

Noninvasive diagnostic studies complement clinical findings. The chest X-ray is a principal tool for evaluating pulmonary parenchymal status and cardiac size, but it is also very helpful for evaluating the significance of a PDA. The X-ray may show progressively increased vascularity (plethora), which may be more noted in the right lung, and a "PDA cardiac configuration" of cardiomegaly with left atrial dilatation, loss of concavity, and left ventricular dilatation (Fig. 3-1A,B). Pulmonary interstitial fluid (pulmonary edema) accumulation may also be present. Cardiac ultrasonography is also helpful in

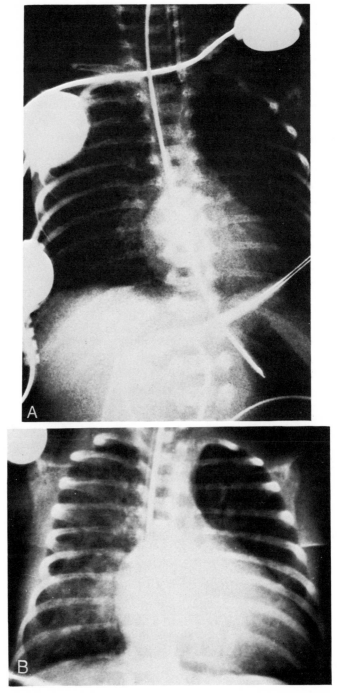

Fig. 3-1.   Chest X-ray changes in neonatal PDA. A. Normal heart size and pulmonary vasculature markings. B. Cardiomegaly with loss of concavity of the pulmonary artery shadow and with increased pulmonary vascular markings, particularly in the right lung.

assessing the presence of a left-to-right shunt at the great vessel level and is indicated with the appearance of a murmur, the presence of CHF, and difficulty in weaning the infant from ventilatory support. On the echocardiogram, the ratio of left atrial dimension to aortic root dimension (LA/Ao ratio) increases as the distensible LA receives an increasing volume of pulmonary venous blood such as occurs in left-to-right ductal shunts (Figure 3-2). The normal ratio is equal to or below 1:1; thus a positive value such as 1.5:1 indicates a significantly enlarged LA consistent with a large ductal shunt. A PDA is not the only cause of an increased LA/Ao ratio; the ratio can also be increased with a ventricular septal defect (VSD) or with hypervolemia in the absence of a shunt. It should be remembered that specific conclusions as to the degree of shunting through the ductus cannot be drawn based on loudness of the murmur or specific size of the LA/Ao ratio on echocardiography. In general, larger LA/Ao ratios are associated with larger shunts, and softer murmurs or no murmurs are associated with smaller shunts, but the largest ductuses may have no murmurs at all. Further, angiography may demonstrate the presence of a PDA despite a normal LA/Ao ratio.[13] Recently, the use of other echocardiographic indices such as systolic time intervals and left ventricular dimensions has been advanced as a means of increasing the sensitivity and specificity of the diagnosis.[14]

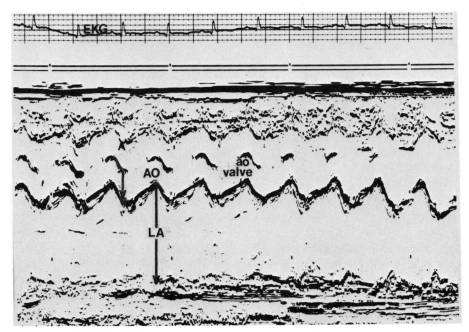

Fig. 3-2.   An M-mode echocardiogram showing increased left atrial-to-aortic root ratio (LA/Ao). Aortic valve motion is clearly seen. This is part of a sweep from the left ventricle through the outflow tract to the aorta. In this example, the LA/Ao is approximately 1.75:1.

Diagnosis of PDA may also be difficult in certain other situations. These include atypical findings (e.g., only a systolic murmur, intermittent murmur, or no murmur) and variability in the degree of left-to-right shunting through the ductus, such as with severe RDS. Although there is a general reluctance to perform extensive catheterization in critically ill newborns, aortic angiography may be necessary in some situations to confirm the presence of a PDA and assess its significance (Fig. 3-3). Other confirmatory tests include contrast echocardiography and radionuclide studies. Current research is attempting to resolve these diagnostic concerns.

Differential diagnosis of PDA involves several disease entities. Ventricular septal defect (VSD) may be indistinguishable from a small PDA in premature newborns by auscultation alone, especially in those whose PDA is manifested only by a systolic murmur, and more direct confirmation may be necessary. In similar fashion to PDA, the VSD murmur may not be heard until PVR decreases. Infants with either a significant PDA or VSD may exhibit CHF, combined ventricular hypertrophy on electrocardiography, and cardiomegaly and increased vascularity on the chest X-ray. In addition to a VSD, the findings

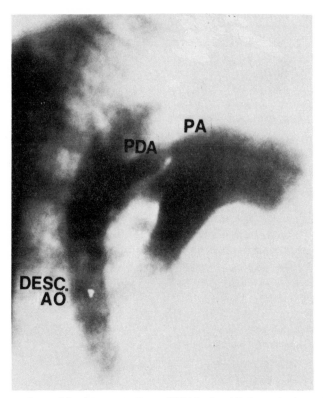

Fig. 3-3. An angiographic demonstration of PDA. In this lateral view, the catheter traverses the PDA after passage through the main pulmonary artery, and the tip is in the descending aorta. Bifurcation of the pulmonary artery is seen.

Table 3-2. Causes of Continuous Murmurs in Infancy

Acyanotic
    Patent ductus arteriosus
    Aortico-pulmonary septal defect
    Coronary arterial fistulae
    Arterio-venous fistulae (systemic or pulmonary)
    Defects of sinus of valsalva
Cyanotic
    Truncus arteriosus
    Postoperative systemic-pulmonary shunt
    Total anomalous pulmonary venous drainage (to right atrium
        or superior vena cava)
    Absent pulmonary valve leaflet syndrome (actually a "to-
        and-fro" murmur)

of a "physiologic" peripheral pulmonary stenosis (PPS) may sometimes mimic a small hemodynamically insignificant PDA. The PPS murmur is early-to-mid-systolic and ejection type, is loudest at the upper left sternal border, and radiates to the axilla and back. It occurs because of either true narrowing in the branch pulmonary arteries or the natural discrepancy in size between the main pulmonary trunk and the branch arteries that may be present in the early postnatal period. Finally, high output states such as tachycardia, anemia, and hyperthermia without evidence of organic heart disease can result in similar auscultative findings.

Thus, auscultative differentiation between the systolic murmurs of PDA, VSD, and PPS may be difficult. However, the following differences may be helpful. The PDA murmur is best heard at the left upper sternal border (LUSB) whereas the VSD murmur is best heard at the left lower sternal border (LLSB), although this difference is not absolute and is further complicated because sounds are easily transmitted over the very small thin chests of premature infants. The small VSD murmur does not radiate to the back. The PPS murmur is soft and is not associated with clinical signs of CHF. Bounding peripheral (e.g., dorsalis pedis) pulses usually occur with PDA as opposed to the other entities. In general, the diagnosis of PDA should be reviewed in the context of other factors affecting the infant, such as the administration of medications. For example, administering respiratory stimulants such as theophylline may result in a significant tachycardia and in some instances even a short systolic murmur. Other causes of continuous murmurs in infancy are noted in Table 3-2.

TREATMENT

Although surgical or pharmacologic closure is often necessary, conservative medical management may help to achieve spontaneous PDA closure because of gradual maturation of the closure mechanism. Depending on the circumstances, however, the infant with hemodynamically significant PDA may be at risk for developing increasing lung damage (bronchopulmonary dysplasia) when ventilator care is prolonged in association with the ductus.[15]

Certain simple measures taken in managing the sick newborn may also be therapeutic in PDA. Maintenance of the hematocrit above 40% increases the oxygen-carrying capacity, thus providing adequate oxygenation to the myocardium and possibly increasing periductal oxygen tension to facilitate ductal closure. Maintenance of the PaO_2 at 60–80 torr may also be necessary. Other measures include using low-solute formula (e.g. Similac PM 60/40 or breast milk), decreasing the caloric expenditure of the infant with gavage rather than nipple feeding, and maintaining a neutral thermal environment. Fluid restriction to a maximum of 100–140 cc/kg/day appears to decrease the incidence of PDA and may rapidly improve symptoms once a PDA has become significant.[16] Careful attention must be paid to maintaining the delicate fluid and electrolyte balance associated with insensible water loss in infants (especially very small prematures) receiving single- and double-light phototherapy. Their fluid requirements may well exceed 150 cc/kg/day for brief periods. Equally important is providing optimal nutritional needs (see Chapter 4). In general, these measures tend to decrease both oxygen consumption and the workload of the heart.

Therapeutic measures may further be necessary to eliminate fluid retention due to CHF. A rapid (10–60 min) and notable diuresis should occur with intravenous furosemide (Lasix) 1–2 mg/kg. A second and double dose may be given if no response is noted in one hour. If maintenance diuretics are indicated, common oral agents include chlorothiazide (Diuril), hydrochlorothiazide (Hydrodiuril), furosemide, and spironolactone (Aldactone), when combined with another agent.

Cardiotonic drugs have been considered the cornerstone of CHF treatment, although recent evidence suggests that digoxin, for example, may be of questionable benefit to the very immature preterm infant with CHF secondary to PDA.[17] Clinical improvement often follows intensive diuretic therapy but is often more difficult to establish after digoxin alone. Reduced blood volume with effective diuresis lowers left-ventricular end diastolic volume (pre-load) and pulmonary venous pressures and favors a decrease in pulmonary edema. Through these mechanisms the workload of the heart decreases, and tolerance to the left-to-right shunt increases.

Experimental findings suggest that the relative indistensibility of the left ventricle in small preterm infants is more a function of myocardial tissue factors than of poor muscle function.[18] Many premature infants demonstrate excellent ventricular muscle function on echocardiography. Thus, the premature infant with a symptomatic PDA may be operating at peak cardiac contractility, and further inotropic support may not be helpful for alleviating symptoms. Of course, if evidence of diminished contractility is available (such as echocardiographic measurements), then inotropic support may indeed be important adjunctive therapy.

The use of digoxin should be tempered with the knowledge that a relatively high drug level of digoxin can be easily achieved among infants with PDA that is associated with RDS.[19] Factors that may contribute to slow clearance of digoxin from serum include hemodynamic disturbances resulting from decreased blood supply to the kidneys and the relative immaturity of renal function.

Medication errors related to administration of the small doses of digoxin can easily occur, and scrupulous attention to medication policies and administration procedures must be followed. Large variations in plasma levels of digoxin with similar dosage regimens have been noted, and thus the truly appropriate dose of digoxin for the premature infant has yet to be unquestionably determined. Currently, dosages of 25–35 µg/kg are administered as total digitalizing doses. Despite these comments, digoxin is still widely used in the premature infant with symptomatic PDA. Proponents of digoxin therapy use it for multiple reasons: (1) a possible positive inotropic response, (2) a direct diuretic effect on the kidneys via an ability to sensitize atrial baroreceptors, and (3) a possible effect to reduce venous return by action on systemic veins. Current research is aimed at further assessing the role of digoxin and other inotropic agents for the premature infant with symptomatic PDA.

When this traditional approach fails to relieve CHF caused by PDA, as manifested by persistent inability to be weaned from the respirator and inability to support adequate spontaneous respiration, by failure to grow because adequate calories cannot be provided, or by intractable apnea or bradycardia, then further therapeutic efforts are necessary.

Until recently the only alternative to continued medical management was surgical ligation of the PDA. This procedure is relatively simple and in most centers surgery itself carries a low mortality risk.[20,21] Ligation is recommended (1) for infants without HMD who develop uncontrollable heart failure, (2) for those who have HMD and deteriorate despite medical therapy, and (3) for those in whom the use of indomethacin is contraindicated or has failed. Currently, some centers are carrying out surgical ligation of the ductus in the premature baby in the intensive care nursery in the first few days of life to mitigate against the complications of prolonged therapy that were noted above. Surgery involves ligation rather than division of the ductus because this structure is often very friable in the premature. The procedure takes 15–20 min. Central and arterial lines are placed, and a general anesthetic agent (e.g., halothane, ketamine, fluroxene, and nitrous oxide) and relaxant is used. The PDA is exposed through a posterolateral position by either a transpleural or extrapleural approach.[22] The latter establishes a plane outside the parietal pleura and permits an excellent view of the PDA and aortic isthmus without entrance into the pleural cavity. This procedure also reduces manipulation of the lung and obviates the need for a chest tube. The PDA and adjacent aorta require careful dissection since the PDA is frequently as large or larger than the transverse aorta. Two ligatures are preferable to one, and blood loss seldom exceeds 15–25 ml.

Within the past 5–7 years, pharmacologic manipulation to close the ductus has been initiated based on knowledge of the role of prostaglandins (PGs) in controlling ductal tone.[9,10,23,24] Prostaglandins are potent smooth-muscle agents present in all tissues. They are derived from essential fatty acids, and at least 14 different biochemically active ones exist. The relative quantities of each PG produced and the level of synthesis activity are species- and organ-dependent. Prostaglandins are classified on the basis of order and discovery (e.g. series PGA, PGB, through the more recently discovered PGI series) plus biologic and chemical behavior. The subscript refers to the fatty-acid precursor compound and thus the number of double bonds in the molecule (e.g., linoleic acid$_1$, arachidonic acid$_2$). Of importance to PDA, compounds in the PGE and PGI series are dilating agents and those in the PGF series are constricting agents (PGE antagonists), of which $PGF_{2\ alpha}$ is the best known. PGI_2 is the major product of arachidonic acid metabolism in the fetal ductus; PGE_2 and $PGF_{2\ alpha}$ are formed in relatively minor amounts. Experimental evidence indicates that PGE_2 is the most potent relaxant formed in the ductus and that it is responsible for maintaining patency of the fetal ductus.[25]

Prostaglandins are released from most organs in response to varied stimuli. They are believed to act as local hormones and possibly influence physiologic reactions by controlling the production of cyclic AMP or cyclic GMP. Calcium may also interact with PG within the cell.

The use of prostaglandin synthetase inhibitors was noted with the discovery of PG's involvement in the inflammatory response mechanism. Prostaglandin synthetase inhibitors (e.g., indomethacin, salicylates) are nonsteroidal anti-inflammatory agents. The major ones tend to be nonselective in their inhibitory effect, and their potential effect at the cellular level may depend on the dominant PG within that system.

Indomethacin (Merck, Sharp & Dohme) was introduced for treatment of rheumatoid arthritis and related disorders because of its anti-inflammatory and antipyretic properties, and possible analgesic effects. Until recently, it was contraindicated for use in children because of the absence of clinical trials. Since 1975, it has been administered frequently under investigational use guidelines to effect closure of PDA in preterm infants.[23,24,26–28] Indomethacin is thought to mediate closure of the PDA by inhibiting the potent smooth-muscle relaxant substances PGI_2 and PGE_2. The drug may induce renal dysfunction and inhibit platelet aggregation and theoretically may also displace bilirubin from albumin. The drug is available in oral and intravenous preparations. Unfortunately there are limitations with both forms. A commercial preparation of oral indomethacin (Indocin®) that is a liquid with uniform composition does not exist; therefore, proper dosimetry and absorption cannot be ensured. Sodium indomethacin (Lyoindocin®), the intravenous form, guarantees delivery of the desired dose but is investigational at this time. Indomethacin is only effective in closing the immature type of PDA.

Premature infants who are candidates for indomethacin therapy demonstrate a large PDA that is unresponsive to aggressive medical management. Administering indomethacin within the first 1–2 postnatal weeks in infants below 33 weeks gestational age at birth is felt to enhance effective ductal closure.[8] Contraindications to use include evidence of renal dysfunction, thrombocytopenia, and confirmation or suspicion of intracranial hemorrhage or necrotizing enterocolitis. Some centers further exclude infants with significant hyperbilirubinemia, sepsis, and meningitis.

Prior to administration of indomethacin, the following laboratory studies should be done: electrolytes, blood urea nitrogen (BUN), creatinine, bilirubin, urinalysis, 12-hr urine for protein when possible; hemoglobin, hematocrit, white blood cell and platelet counts; test for occult blood in the stool, and blood-gas analysis.

In the absence of contraindications, indomethacin (0.2–0.3 mg/kg/dose) is given orally through a nasogastric tube or intravascularly. It may be given via an umbilical artery line if the placement is below L_4 to insure drug dilution before the first pass through the kidneys. The rate of delivery should be slow, over 1–5 min per dose. The frequency and time intervals depend on individual preference and the clinical picture, and intervals have varied from every 6, 8, or 12 hrs to 24 hrs apart until a total dose of 0.6 mg/kg has been administered. Meticulous serial assessments of cardiopulmonary status and clinical and laboratory measures to detect renal function, bleeding, bilirubin problems (if believed necessary), intracranial hemorrhage, and necrotizing enterocolitis are essential during the course of treatment.

Side effects are generally dose dependent and occur with more frequency and severity with larger doses. The most significant side effect involves abnormal renal function. Oliguria is transient and usually lasts 12–24 hours; however, more prolonged reduction in urine output has been reported. Anuria rarely occurs, but renal dysfunction has been reported.[29] BUN and creatinine may increase moderately, especially in fluid restricted infants treated with diuretics. Preexisting renal pathology may be a factor in the development of renal side effects. No correlations can yet be made between potential inhibition of platelet function by indomethacin and an increased incidence of intracranial hemorrhage or of gastrointestinal bleeding and necrotizing enterocolitis.

Evidence of closure as the result of indomethacin may be dramatic and occur in a few hours, or it may take several days. Closure may not always be complete, but a sufficient degree of constriction may occur to reduce shunting and produce clinical improvement. Some investigators believe that it is not necessary to demand immediate complete closure of the ductus by indomethacin but that success is represented by marked improvement of symptoms and that more complete closure can then occur within several days. Subsequent recurrence with cardiopulmonary difficulties occurs in many infants after indomethacin therapy and may warrant a second treatment regimen in the absence of contraindications. In the event of contraindications or if indomethacin is unsuccessful—as has been reported—the infant may be a candidate for surgical ligation even after a course of drug therapy.[30]

COMPLICATIONS AND RELATIONSHIP TO THERAPY

The earliest complication of PDA in the neonate is CHF. Uncontrollable CHF may be associated with fluid and electrolyte imbalance, nutritional deficiency, and failure of the infant to be weaned from ventilator assistance; this dependence leads to prolonged respiratory support, which may be associated with bronchopulmonary dysplasia. Intracranial hemorrhage, a primary cause of death in infants with HMD (see Chapter 1), may occur more frequently with PDA than is currently suspected.

Secondary complications may occur in other organs when a large left-to-right shunt compromises blood flow to the descending aorta. These include gut ischemia, alterations in renal blood flow, and central-nervous-system effects. A postulated relationship between the development of necrotizing enterocolitis and the presence of a large left-to-right shunt via a PDA that creates a "mesenteric steal" has been proposed. Other common findings are decreased urine output and metabolic acidosis.

Data from a 1–year follow-up study of a group of babies in which 55% of the infants had symptomatic PDA and were compared with age-matched controls without PDA indicated the following morbidity:[31] approximately 75% of the babies with PDA had mild-to-severe neurologic abnormalities including low Bailey scores, seizures, decreased hearing, hypotonia, and abnormal Denver Developmental Screening Tests (DDSTs) whereas 44% of the babies without PDA had abnormal neurologic follow-up. Of special concern was that three infants who had prolonged PDA, one of whom required surgical PDA ligation, died of sudden infant death syndrome. Other, more recent studies, have demonstrated effective closure of PDA with varying courses and doses of indomethacin in infants with RDS and that closure in these instances results in less morbidity and mortality from the underlying RDS.[26,27] The results of a multicenter, collaborative study involving over 1300 premature infants are pending; it is hoped that these results will further delineate the efficacy of indomethacin and also the relationship of PDA to other medical problems of the critically ill premature infant.

When considering the use of prostaglandin synthetase inhibitors such as indomethacin for treating PDA, one must weigh the risks of such therapy against the benefits of PDA closure and the risks of surgical ligation. In one randomized study that contrasted early surgical ligation versus standard medical management not including indomethacin and in which long-term follow-up was not mentioned, advocates of early ligation cited the following benefits: earlier successful extubation (5 days); earlier age at which at least 80 kcal/kg could be provided gastrointestinally; and an absolute reduction in cost per patient.[32] Proponents of indomethacin have not detected any late complications with reference to psychomotor development, vision, neurologic function, resistance to infection, bleeding tendency, or renal function in treated infants followed for periods varying up to 11 months.[33] The advantages of avoiding surgery include a spared thoracotomy, reduced cost and duration of hospitalization, and avoidance of the risks and anxieties associated with surgery and anesthesia.

Currently, the final results are not available regarding which type of therapy is best with respect to both immediate and long-term outcomes, although several major studies are in progress. Data that specifically addresses these issues will soon be forthcoming from the national collaborative study on using indomethacin for closure of the ductus arteriosus. Medical therapy that is prolonged while one waits for the PDA to close spontaneously can be problematic and associated with an increased risk of chronic lung disease and other sequelae. Indomethacin is effective in some infants, but the PDA may reopen. Also, neither all the immediate nor the long-term side effects of the drug are known. Surgery effectively ligates the ductus but carries its own risks and benefits. Many authorities consider that the expense accompanying the increased hospitalization required for infants who undergo surgical ligation of the ductus as compared with those who receive indomethacin provides abundant justification for pursuing nonsurgical methods to minimize or alleviate this common problem. In most instances, one should consider the clinical circumstances such as the severity of the infant's condition and the associated medical problems when deciding on the most appropriate course of therapy.

THE ROLE OF THE DUCTUS IN CERTAIN FORMS OF CONGENITAL HEART DISEASE

In contrast to the previously described clinical situations in which closure of the ductus arteriosus is the desired outcome of medical or surgical intervention, in certain instances maintenance of ductal patency is the aim of therapy.

In particular, newborn infants with obstruction to pulmonary blood flow depend on ductal patency and right-to-left shunting via the ductus for maintenance of adequate systemic oxygenation. The cardiac lesions associated with this clinical problem are noted in Table 3-3. In these forms of heart disease, the ductus arteriosus may be longer and narrower than in children with normal cardiac anatomy, perhaps because of altered intrauterine flow patterns, and thus even relatively small degrees of constriction after birth can result in significant reduction of ductal flow.[34] It is noteworthy that the ductus can constrict in these infants even though systemic arterial oxygen saturation is low. The precise details of the mechanism of closure in such situations are not known.

As has been noted above, it is currently thought that the prostaglandins are important in regulating ductal patency *in utero* and that the acknowledged fall in circulating prostaglandins after delivery is related to constriction of the ductus arteriosus. Specifically, PGE_1 and PGE_2 have been identified as dilators of isolated ductus arteriosus strips of fetal lambs. PGE_1 has been used in several clinical trials to maintain ductal patency and hence pulmonary blood flow, and

Table 3-3. Ductal-Dependent Congenital Heart Lesions

A. Ductal-dependent pulmonary blood flow
   Pulmonary atresia ⎱ intact septum
   Tricuspid atresia ⎰
   Critical pulmonary stenosis

B. Ductal-dependent systemic blood flow
   Coarctation of the aorta
   Aortic arch interruption
   Hypoplastic left heart syndrome

thereby increase arterial oxygen saturation in these forms of cyanotic heart disease.[35,36]

The indications for use of prostaglandins, notably PGE_1, in these conditions include progressive arterial desaturation and worsening acidemia. The cardiac diagnosis should be established by cardiac catheterization and cineangiography. Although most centers currently seek to infuse PGE_1 through a catheter positioned with its orifice at the aortic origin of the ductus, many cases of successful ductal manipulation have been accomplished even with peripheral intravenous PGE_1 administration. Doses range from 0.05–0.10 µg/kg/min. In most infants, improvement in arterial PO_2 is apparent within minutes, with peak results seen at 30–45 min. With the improving status of tissue oxygenation, acidemia is also relieved, and the improved clinical picture generally persists for as long as the prostaglandin perfusion is maintained. The primary aim of this therapy is to stabilize the infant or to improve the clinical status of a severely ill infant until surgical palliation can be arranged. In fact, available clinical data indicate that surgical results are improved when the infant has undergone a period of stabilization on PGE_1 infusion.[37]

In certain circumstances, prostaglandin infusion may be carried out not to maintain ductal patency *per se* but for a vasodilatory effect on the pulmonary vascular bed. Much current investigation is focusing on use of these agents for treating infants with so-called "persistent fetal circulation syndrome", in which pulmonary blood flow is restricted by abnormally elevated pulmonary vascular resistance despite normal intracardiac anatomy. Whereas results with PGE_1 and prostacyclin (PGI) have been disappointing thus far, recent experimental data have suggested a possible role for PGD in this situation.[38] However, further careful evaluation is required in clinical situations to clarify these treatment options. It should be noted, in view of earlier discussions in this chapter, that one demonstrated etiologic consideration for babies with persistent postnatal elevation of pulmonary vascular resistance (PFC syndrome) is intrauterine closure of the ductus arteriosus as occurs in mothers ingesting either indomethacin or other prostaglandin inhibitors such as aspirin.[39]

In addition to clinical problems of reduced pulmonary blood flow, ductal manipulation with the use of prostaglandins can also be beneficial for infants with interruptions of systemic blood flow (Table 3-3B). In these situations, descending aortic flow is dependent either on blood shunted from the pulmonary artery to it via the ductus or on the presence of the ductus ampulla, which allows blood to pass around the posterior shelf that restricts the aortic lumen.[40]

These infants usually do not manifest marked hypoxemia, although arterial PO_2 may be reduced below normal. Congestive heart failure with pulmonary edema is the principle clinical presentation. At times, this may be overwhelming and the infant may be in extremis with nearly unpalpable peripheral pulses, ashen appearance, diminished urine output, and marked tachypnea. Metabolic acidosis can be greater than that seen in any other neonatal disease and the picture confused with septicemia or congenital organic acidosis.

Once diagnosis is established at cardiac catheterization, PGE_1 can be infused as noted above. Immediate improvement in descending aortic pressure and flow is noted and reflected in improved mean arterial pressure and increased urinary output. Eventually, improvement in pH and arterial blood gas status will be evident.

Thus, manipulation of the ductus arteriosus can be aimed at patency in addition to closure. Of course, the clinical situations are vastly different, but personnel involved in the critical care of infants should be aware of both options.

IMPLICATIONS FOR NURSING

Survival of critically ill infants may be directly related to the skill of the personnel providing the care in the neonatal intensive care unit. Since a wide variability in providing such care exists among neonatal centers, recognition and treatment of infants with PDA associated with RDS and of those with congenital heart lesions that are dependent on a patent ductus arteriosus may not be optimal. Factors that are going to further affect this situation are the increasing numbers of surviving premature infants and the decreasing ratio of experienced house staff and neonatal fellows per infant.[41] This will necessitate increased application of clinical assessment skills in the staff that has the closest contact with the infant. Therefore, it is important for critical care nurses to have a clear understanding of the physiologic concepts and the diagnostic and physical assessment skills. This expertise will facilitate intelligent assessment of clinical findings, early diagnosis, prompt intervention, and evaluation of treatment.

The remaining discussion will focus on PDA that is associated with RDS because it occurs more frequently than ductus-dependent heart lesions.

Variability of Signs and Importance of Ausculation

The goal of nursing intervention is to prevent or minimize the effects of PDA. Preventing PDA is not always possible, but minimizing its effects often is. Anticipating the infants likely to develop symptomatic PDA and the timing of its development is relatively straight-foreward, as discussed above in the section on assessment parameters. However, extreme variability of signs (murmurs, pulses, pulse pressure, perfusion states, cyanosis, work of breathing) can occur among infants and also within the same infant from hour to hour and even minute to minute and can create problems for physicians who examine the infants only two or three times per day. Furthermore, their conclusions may vary with those of other physicans who examine the infants at different times (and, sometimes, even at the same time). These discrepancies may be appropriate because of the rapidly changing pulmonary vascular resistance and hemodynamics.

Unless careful auscultation is performed frequently by an experienced person, especially in infants with HMD who require ventilatory assistance via an endotracheal tube, the murmur can easily be missed. Neonatal critical care nurses and neonatal critical care nurse practitioners (NCCNPs) can develop their auscultation skills and make a vital contribution to hourly management of these infants and thereby positively affect their clinical course. The ability to identify the point of maximum impulse and the presence or absence of a murmur is important. The further ability to identify S_1 and S_2 heart sounds and the presence of a gallop and to differentiate between systolic and diastolic murmurs develops only with practice. A skilled nurse clinician can recognize the type of murmur and its meaning, collaborate through reporting these findings, and facilitate early diagnosis and treatment.

Nursing Interventions

Nursing interventions to prevent or minimize PDA are directed to eliminating demands that increase oxygen and caloric consumption. Chapter 1 mentions nursing interventions to decrease stressors and also to provide support for the high-risk infant, and this chapter has discussed medical preventive and therapeutic measures in the section on treatment options. The two approaches are complementary. However, the sine qua non is well-planned, coordinated care.

Physical assessment should be done at least once each shift (more often if needed) in infants suspected of developing a PDA or in those who already have a PDA. It should preferably be done when the infant is at rest and before care is begun. Skillful assessment can be done gently, quickly, and efficiently, with minimal disturbance to the infant. The nurse should coordinate this examination with other personnel who may want to observe or participate in it. Assessments should be recorded and significant findings communicated promptly to appropriate members of the team. Heart sounds and murmurs should be documented descriptively and/or graphically (Fig. 3-4). This organized approach fosters trust, instructs, prevents random examinations by different examiners, and minimizes disturbances to the infant.

The following considerations to facilitate evaluation of the infant are least obvious to individuals who do limited physical assessment and interpretation of chest X-rays. These considerations improve accessibility to the infant, improve the quality of the examination, and decrease needless and unpleasant stimuli such as those that lead to skin trauma and breakdown.

Infant ECG electrodes should be used and placed away from the anterior chest (especially the left infraclavicular area and the third to fourth interspaces at the mid-clavicular lines bilaterally) and away from the right upper quadrant of the abdomen. Improper lead placement obscures cardiac auscultation, radiographic evaluation of the lung fields, and palpation of the liver. Since many infants are transported to regional centers, the initial application of the electrodes should be done by the referral hospital. Otherwise, the transport team should apply them properly. Additional factors that interfere with evaluation

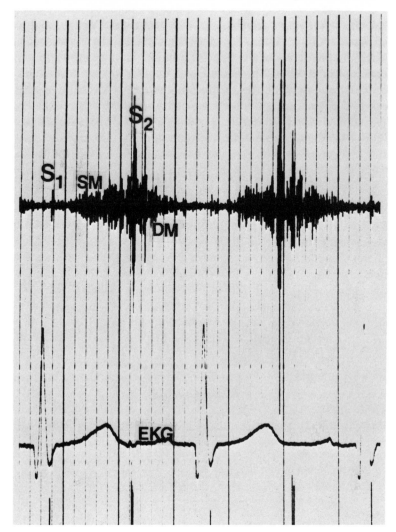

Fig. 3-4. A phonocardiogram of a continuous murmur associated with PDA. The tracing was recorded from the upper left precordium. S_1, first heart sound; S_2, second heart sound; SM, systolic component; DM, diastolic component; EKG, simultaneous electrocardiogram.

are the excessive application of tape associated with umbilical lines, temperature probes, and $TcPO_2$ electrodes, and also the placement and direction of such items in these areas. Ideal electrode and probe placement may not always be possible. Nonetheless, special attention can prevent limited access to a complete physical examination and interference with an echocardiographic study. In this way, unnecessary repetition of chest X-rays because of obscured lung regions and cardiac silhouette can also be avoided.

When clinical findings indicate the need for a chest X-ray, echocardiogram, or ECG, the nurse should try to coordinate the time of the study with the technician to benefit the infant best and then should assist the technician. Chest X-rays are most effective when they are columnated (when the infant's position is non-rotated) and when the film is not hampered by electrodes, lead wires, and other items. Assisting the technician can help prevent temperature loss, needless disturbance of the infant, and unreliable studies. Arranging a time with the technician is considerate, especially when there is only one available technician who generally must fit the infant into an already busy schedule.

CONCLUSION

Ongoing evaluation of the infant's response to the nursing and medical plan is essential to provide optimal care. Current research is contributing much to the knowledge and care of PDA—especially that associated with RDS and with ductus-dependent cardiac lesions. Neonatal critical care nurses have a responsibility to upgrade their knowledge based on current research findings. They also have an important role in the evaluation of these clinical problems, in their prevention and early detection, and in prompt and appropriate intervention. Collaborative efforts among medical personnel contribute to excellence of care and are expected to improve the outcome for the infant and the family.

REFERENCES

1. Barnard ED: Discussion on the significance of continuous murmurs in the first few days of life. Proc Roy Soc Med 52:77–78, 1959
2. Neal WA, Bessinger FB, Hunt CE, et al.: Patent ductus arteriosus complicating respiratory distress syndrome. J Pediatr 86:127, 1975
3. Siassi B, Bianco C, Cabal LA, et al.: Incidence and clinical features of patent ductus arteriosus in low-birth weight infants. A prospective analysis of 150 consecutively born infants. Pediatrics 57:347, 1976
4. Kitterman JA, Edmunds LH Jr, Gregory GA, et al.: Patent ductus arteriosus in premature infants: incidence, relation to pulmonary disease and management. N Engl J Med 287:473, 1972.
5. Bell EF, Warburton D, Stonestreet BS, et al.: Effect of fluid administration on the development of symptomatic patent ductus arteriosus and congestive heart failure in premature infants. N Eng J Med 302:598, 1980
6. Thibleault DW, Emmanouildes GG, Nelson RJ, et al.: Patent ductus arteriosus complicating the respiratory distress syndrome in preterm infants. J Pediatr 86:120, 1975
7. Rudolph AM: The role of the ductus arteriosus in the fetus and postnatal circulatory changes. In: The Ductus Arteriosus, Proceedings of the Seventy-Fifth Ross Conference on Pediatric Research, ed. Heymann MA, Rudolph AM. Ross Laboratories, Columbus, Ohio, 1978, p 116
8. Gittenberger-de-Groot AC, Van Ertbruggen I, Moulaert AJMG, et al.: The ductus arteriosus in the preterm infant: histologic and clinical observations. J Pediatr 96:88, 1980

9. Clyman RI: Ontogeny of the ductus arteriosus responses to prostaglandins and inhibitors of their synthesis. Semin Perinatol 4:115, 1980

10. Kirkpatrick SE, Printz MP, Friedman WF: Prostaglandins in the fetal ductus arteriosus. Pediatr Res 11:394, 1979

11. Gittenberger-de-Groot AC: Persistent ductus arteriosus: most probably a primary congenital malformation. Br Heart J 39:610, 1977

12. Rudolph AM: The pre- and postnatal pulmonary circulation. In: Congenital Diseases of the Heart, ed. Rudolph AM. Chicago, Yearbook Med Pub, 1974, pp 29–48

13. Valdes-Cruz LM, Dudell G: Specificity and accuracy of echocardiographic and clinical criteria for diagnosis of patent ductus arteriosus in fluid restricted infants. J Pediatr 98:298, 1981

14. Johnson GL, Desai N, Cottrill CM et al.: Echocardiographic systolic time intervals in premature infants with patent ductus arteriosus. Pediatr Cardiol 1:103, 1979

15. Northway WJ, Rosen RC, Porter DY: Pulmonary disease following respiratory therapy of hyaline membrane disease. N Engl J Med 276:357, 1967

16. Stevenson JG: Fluid administration in the association of patent ductus arteriosus complicating respiratory distress syndrome. J Pediatr 90:257, 1977

17. White RD, Lietman PS: Commentary: a reappraisal of digitalis for infants with left-to-right shunts and "heart failure". J Pediatr 92:867, 1978

18. Friedman WF: The intrinsic physiologic properties of the developing heart. In: Neonatal Heart Disease. eds. Friedman WF, Lesch M, and Sonnenbleck EH. Grune and Stratton, New York 1973, p 21

19. Rogers MC, Willerson JT, Goldblatt A, et al.: Serum digoxin concentrations in the human fetus, neonate, and infant. N Engl J Med 287:1010, 1972

20. Murphy DA, Outerbridge E, Stern L, et al.: Management of premature infants with patent ductus arteriosus. J Thorac Cardiovasc Surg 67:221, 1974

21. Edmunds LH Jr, Gregory GA, Heymann MA, et al.: Surgical closure of the ductus arteriosus in premature infants. Circulation 48:856, 1973

22. Clark DR, Paton BC, Gay WL, et al.: Patent ductus arteriosus ligation and respiratory distress syndrome in premature infants. Ann Thorac Surg 22:138, 1976

23. Friedman WJ, Huschklan MJ, Printz MP, et al.: Pharmacologic closure of patent ductus arteriosus in the premature infant. N Eng J Med 295:526, 1976

24. Heymann MA, Rudolph AM, Silverman NH: Closure of the ductus arteriosus in premature infants by inhibition of prostaglandin synthesis. N Engl J Med 295:530, 1976

25. Clyman RI, Mauray F, Roman C, et al.: PGE_2 is a more potent vasodilator of the lamb ductus arteriosus than is either PGI_2 or 6 Keto $F_{1\alpha}$. Prostaglandins 16:259, 1978

26. Yanagi RM, Wilson A, Newfeld EA, et al.: Indomethacin treatment for symptomatic patent ductus arteriosus: a double-blind control study. Pediatrics 67:647, 1981

27. Yeh RF, Luken SA, Thalji A, et al.: Intravenous indocin therapy in premature infants with PDA: a double-blind control study. J Pediatr 98:137, 1981

28. Halliday HL, Huata T, Brady LP: Indomethacin therapy for large patent ductus arteriosus in the very low birth weight infant: results and complications. Pediatrics 64:154, 1979

29. Winther L, Printz MP, Mendoza SA, et al.: The influence of indomethacin on neonatal renal function. Pediatr Res 11: 4 (abstr), 1977

30. Neal WA, Kyle LM, Mullet MD: Failure of indomethacin therapy to induce closure of patent ductus arteriosus in premature infants with respiratory distress syndrome. J Pediatr 91:621, 1977

31. Merritt TA, DeSessa TG, Feldman BH, et al.: Closure of the patent ductus arteriosus with ligation and indomethacin: a consecutive experience. J Pediatr 96:639, 1978

32. Cotton RB. Randomized trial of early closure of symptomatic PDA. In The Ductus Arteriosus. Proceedings of the Seventy-Fifth Ross Conference on Pediatric research. ed. Heymann MA, Rudolph AM. Columbus, Ohio, Ross Laboratories, 1978, p 176.

33. Friedman WF, Heymann MA, Rudolph AM: Commentary—new thoughts on an old problem—patent ductus arteriosus in the premature infant. J Pediatr 90:338, 1977

34. Heymann MA, Rudolph AM: Neonatal manipulation: patent ductus arteriosus. In: Pediatric Cardiovascular Disease, ed. Engle MA, Cardiovascular Clinics 11/2. Philadelphia, FA Davis, 1981, pp 301–310

35. Olley PM, Coceani F, Bodach E: E-type prostaglandins: a new emergency therapy for certain cyanotic congenital heart malformations. Circulation 53:728, 1976

36. Lewis AB, Takahashi M, Lurie PR: Administration of prostaglandin E_1 in neonates with critical congenital cardiac defects. J Pediatr 93:481, 1978

37. Olley PM, Coceani F, Rowe RD: Role of prostaglandin E_1 and E_2 in the management of neonatal heart disease. In: Advances in Prostaglandin and Thromboxane Research. Prostaglandins and Perinatal Medicine. vol 4, eds. Coceani F, and Olley PM, New York, Raven Press 1978, p 345

38. Soiffer SJ, Moren FC, Roman C, et al.: Prostaglandin D_2 (PGD_2) decreases hypoxic pulmonary hypertension in newborn lambs. Pediatr Res 15:682, 1981 (abstr)

39. Levin DL, Fixler DE, Morriss FC, et al.: Morphologic analysis of the pulmonary vascular bed in infants exposed in utero to prostaglandin synthetase inhibitors. J Pediatr 92:478, 1978

40. Talner NS, Berman, MA: Postnatal development of obstruction in coarctation of the aorta: role of the ductus arteriosus. Pediatrics 56:562, 1975

41. Sheldon RE, Dominiak PS: The expanding role of the neonatal nurse. In: The Expanding Role of the Nurse in the Neonatal Intensive Care, eds. Sheldon RE and Dominiak PS. New York, Grune and Stratton, 1980, p 7

4 | Nutritional Management of the Critically Ill Neonate

Mildred D. Boettcher
Gilberto R. Pereira

Meeting the nutritional requirements of critically ill neonates has always been difficult because their clinical status is constantly changing and their ability to regulate fluids and metabolize nutrients is limited. Whereas the full-term neonate is fully capable of developing several physiologic functions crucial for the transition from intra- to extrauterine life, the premature infant is only partially capable of developing these adaptive functions. The purpose of this chapter is to provide nurses with the knowledge necessary to recognize the initial nutritional difficulties of sick neonates during this period of physiologic adaptation, monitor the intake of nutrients, and assess nutritional deficiencies. Physiologic principles of metabolism of infancy are presented with guidelines for nutritional assessment to aid in the selection of the most appropriate nutritional (enteral and/or parenteral) intervention.

It is well recognized that the field of nutrition has for many years been neglected from the training curriculum of health care professionals. It is now accepted that maintaining patients in good nutritional status is an important goal that will most certainly improve the overall medical care provided to sick neonates.

IMPORTANCE OF ADEQUATE NUTRITION

In recent years, interest concerning the provision of optimal nutrition to high-risk neonates has been renewed. Reasons for this renewal include the increasing survival of these infants, especially of small premature infants,[1] and the adverse effects that malnutrition imposes on many organs and physiologic functions. The well-publicized studies of Stock and Smythe[2] and of Winick and associates[3-5] have documented impaired growth of several organs in both animals and humans affected by malnutrition. The organs more severely affected were the ones in active phase of growth at the time the malnutrition occurred. Winick's work disclosed an important correlation between inadequate nutrition and decreased DNA content of various organs including the brain and delineated the ultimate effects of malnutrition on neurologic development. In addition, this work has shown that serial increments in head circumference reflect linear brain growth and are a sensitive indicator of nutritional status.

The adverse influence of malnutrition on the immunologic status is another topic worthy of special attention because of the abnormal defense mechanisms of neonates. These faulty mechanisms are particularly depressed in low-birth-weight (LBW) infants and include (1) a deficient supply of neutrophils,[6] (2) decreased bacteriocidal activity of leukocytes,[7,8] (3) impaired chemotaxis of neutrophils and monocytes,[9,10] and (4) a deficient supply of complement.[11] Superimposed malnutrition further increases the susceptibility of these infants to bacterial infections.

In 1972, Lubchenco[12] reported that changes in nursery policies such as institution of routine intravenous administration of dextrose and early initiation of feeding in premature infants were accompanied by decreased morbidity and improved long-term outcome of premature infants. More recently, the importance of improving nutritional care has been recognized as a crucial factor in reducing surgical morbidity and mortality[13] and in successfully weaning patients off mechanical ventilation.[14]

NUTRITIONAL ASSESSMENT AND PHYSIOLOGIC PRINCIPLES—IMPLICATIONS FOR NURSING PRACTICE

Inspection

Nutritional assessment should begin as soon as the infant is admitted to the Neonatal Intensive Care Unit. General physical inspection provides a variety of important observations that reflect nutritional status. Lethargy is observed in most infants who receive inadequate calories, and overall decreased activity is a constant finding in protein–calorie malnutrition. An examination of the skin, hair, lips, mucous membranes, and extremities may show abnormalities compatible with specific nutritional deficiencies (Table 4-1).

Table 4-1. Clinical Signs of Nutritional Deficits

Area of Exam	Clinical Signs	Deficiency
Hair	falling out lack of luster lack of color	essential fatty acid deficiency (EFAD) zinc, copper
Skin	petechiae, purpura scrotal dermatitis pellagrous dermatitis acrodermatitis and pigmentation	zinc, copper
Face	nasolabial seborrhea	zinc
Eyes	spectacle dull, dry conjunctiva	biotin vitamin A
Lips	bleeding gums angular scars cheilosis	ascorbic acid B-complex, iron, protein
Tongue	glossitis edema	niacin, riboflavin, B_{12} folate, iron
Glands	parotic enlargement thyroid enlargement	protein ascorbic acid iodine
Extremities	dependent edema muscle wasting	hypoalbuminemia vitamin E caloric malnutrition
Skeleton	bowed legs bossing of skull deformities	vitamin D osteomalacia

From: Sandstead HH, Pearson WN: Clinical evaluation of nutritional status. In: Modern Nutrition in Health and Disease. eds. Goodhart R, Shils ME. edn 5, 1976, p 674–675

Anthropometrics

Because growth is so rapid in early infancy, anthropometric changes that reflect growth are commonly used as parameters to assess nutritional status. Serial determination of weight, length, and head circumference are widely recorded in most nurseries to make adjustments in the intake of nutrients by neonates. It is a nursing responsibility to obtain accurate daily weights and weekly lengths and head circumferences in all neonates. Length should be measured with the infant in a supine position with the head firmly held against a vertical surface, the knees stretched, and the soles of the feet held against a vertical sliding board. Head circumference is measured with a non-stretchable tape firmly placed on the maximal occipital prominence around to the area just above the eyebrows. These measurements should be plotted weekly on growth charts that combine standards for both intrauterine (premature) and extrauterine (full-term) growth. Although most sick premature infants do not grow

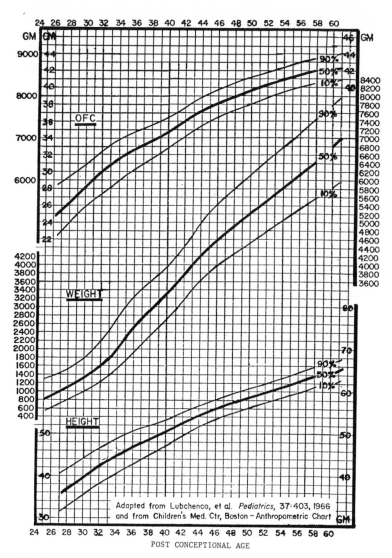

Fig. 4-1.   Combined Intrauterine-Neonatal Growth Chart for Height, Weight, and OFC.

at rates that are comparable with fetal growth, these parameters are regarded by the Committee on Nutrition of the American Academy of Pediatrics as the standards by which nutritional requirements for LBW infants should be calculated.[15] The Lubchenco and Babson growth charts (Figs. 4-1,2) provide guidelines for assessing growth in neonates. Whereas both charts include a preterm section, each chart has different advantages. Lubchenco's chart is more useful for the hospitalized infant because it permits weekly recording of variations in growth parameters for 5 months after the term date. Babson's chart is more suitable for long-term follow-up because it allows recording of growth parameters for 12 months after the term date. However, because the Babson graph is presented at 2-week intervals preterm and 4-week intervals postterm, weekly variations are difficult to assess. Triceps-skinfold thickness (TSF), a valuable parameter for assessing nutrition in older children and adults has not yet been standardized for LBW infants. Mean ± SD triceps skinfold values for fullterm infants at 1 month of age, as reported by Tanner et al.,[16] were 7.4 ± 0.52 mm for boys and 7.5 ± 0.46 mm for girls. At The Children's Hospital of Philadelphia serial arm circumference and TSF measurements were performed on a sample of 13 critically ill premature infants born between 30–32 weeks gestation with birth weight less than 1500 g. These measurements were recorded from 30–32 weeks post-conceptional age and are summarized in Table 4-2.

Biochemical Parameters

Serum protein levels are useful indicators of nutritional status in children and adults. In premature infants, cord values of total serum protein and albumin have been shown to increase progressively with gestational age. According to

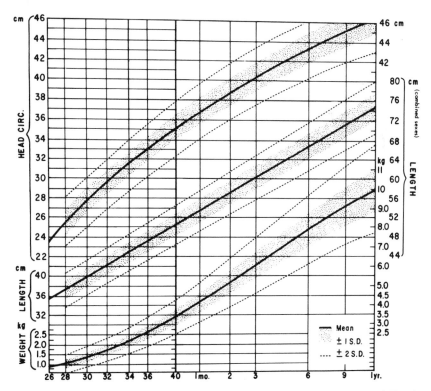

Fig. 4-2. Growth Record for Infants in Relation to Gestational Age and Fetal and Infant Norms. From Babson SG, Benda GI: J. Pediatr. 89:814, 1976.

Table 4-2. Arm Circumference (AC) and Triceps Skinfold Thickness (TSF) in 13 Premature Infants Followed from Birth to Discharge

Post-conceptional Age (weeks)	AC (cm)		TSF (mm)	
	Mean	Range	Mean	Range
32 (8)*	5.6	5.1–6.25	2.4	2.0–3.0
33 (4)	6.1	5.5–6.75	3.1	2.4–4.4
34 (1)	6.3	5.8–7.40	2.9	2.0–4.5
35	6.5	5.9–7.20	3.2	2.6–4.7
36	6.8	5.8–7.40	3.1	2.7–3.5
37	7.2	6.2–8.00	3.3	2.3–4.0
38	7.5	7.0–8.10	3.3	2.5–4.2
39	8.0	7.3–9.10	3.6	3.2–4.2
40	7.9	7.4–8.60	3.9	3.0–5.0

* ( ), number of premature infants born. Data provided by Sharon Moskowitz, R.D., M.S., Clinical Nutritionist and Instructor in Pediatrics, The Children's Hospital of Philadelphia.

Bland[17] mean cord levels of total proteins vary from 3.5 mg/dl at 28 weeks of gestation to 6 mg/dl at term. However, we observed in a previous study of 53 premature infants followed from birth through discharge that levels of total serum protein did not increase significantly from birth, in spite of adequate caloric intake and appropriate growth rates.[18] We therefore concluded that total serum proteins did not seem to be a sensitive indicator of the nutritional status in premature infants.

Recently, several investigators have studied the variation in serum levels of retinol binding protein and pre-albumin as indicators of nutritional status.[19,20] Because these two proteins have a shorter half-life and smaller pool size than albumin, it has been postulated that they might be a more sensitive index of protein adequacy. Presently, pre-albumin levels are being studied in our intensive care unit as part of nutritional monitoring protocol for premature infants. Preliminary data of this study showed that mean ± SD cord levels of pre-albumin in 12 premature infants born from 25–37 weeks gestational age were lower than fullterm values (8.5 ± 2.3 mg/dl for premature vs. 12.0 ± 3.9 mg/dl for term infants) (Moskowitz S, Watkins J, Spitzer AR, Pereira GR; personal communication). In premature infants studied from birth to term age, pre-albumin levels dropped markedly after birth and increased progressively with age. These serum values ranged from 3.5–16.4 mg/dl and correlated with protein and caloric intake. Levels of pre-albumin below 12 mg/dl identified those infants receiving inadequate amounts of proteins and calories. However, further data are needed before this nutritional parameter can be incorporated into routine nutritional monitoring.

Nitrogen balance studies have been used extensively for several decades as a definitive method to assess anabolism and catabolism of ingested proteins and as a standard method to assess nutritional status. Positive and negative nitrogen balance are easily measured by calculating the difference between nitrogen ingested from protein and that lost in urine and stools. However, the technical difficulties in accurately collecting all urine and stool specimens over a 24-hr period in critically ill infants makes its application for routine use less desirable. It was recently reported that 3-methylhystidine, an inert catabolite that results from skeletal muscle protein breakdown, could serve as a valuable marker for assessing protein malnutrition in adults and children.[21] In 1979, Ballard et al.[22] reported on the urinary levels of 3-methylhystidine in 36 premature infants with birth weights varying from 0.6–1.2 kg. Daily urinary levels of that catabolite ranged from 1.7–6.2 mMoles/kg and had a highly significant inverse correlation with nitrogen balance. If the excretion rates of 3-methylhystidine prove to be constant throughout the day, spot measurements of this metabolite may become a practical test for nutritional monitoring of premature infants.

ENERGY AND FLUID THERAPY

Energy Requirements

In the absence of external work, energy balance of the whole body may be defined as follows:

Energy intake = energy expenditure + energy excreted + energy stored

Energy Intake

In principle, gross energy intake from ingestion of foods is always greater than the ultimate amount of energy available to the body. This difference results from the fact that most feedings are not completely absorbed and metabolized. This is especially true in the premature infant because of the significant degree of malabsorption of ingested fats, carbohydrates, and proteins. Another important factor is that there are variabilities in the caloric content of breast milk that depend on the length of gestation, time of lactation, and maternal individuality. The energy available from metabolizing carbohydrate, fat, and protein is calculated as 4, 9, and 4 Cal/g, respectively.

Energy Expenditures

Energy expenditures include the energy utilized for all physiologic functions of the body such as cardiorespiratory activity, digestion, physical activity, temperature maintenance, and growth. Stressful conditions such as hypothermia, hyperthermia, and respiratory distress (which increases the work of breathing) significantly increase energy requirements. Mainstays in the nursing care of infants with these conditions include providing an environment that minimizes heat loss and physical activity and respiratory support as needed (see Chapter 1).

Energy Excreted

Because of the immaturity of their enzymatic processes the amount of energy lost in urine and stools is significantly increased in LBW infants. For

Table 4-3. Estimate of Caloric Expenditure During the Neonatal Period

Expenditure	Cal/kg/24 hr
Minimal (non-growing) expenditure	
Resting	50
Intermittent activity	0–15
Occasional cold stress	0–10
Total	50–75
Additional expenditure with growth	
Specific dynamic action	10
Fecal losses	10
Growth	25
Total	45
Total caloric expenditure	95–120

From Winters RW: The Body Fluids in Pediatrics. In: Maintenance Fluid Therapy, Winters RW ed., Boston, Little Brown, 1973, p 267

example, fats are incompletely absorbed by the gastrointestinal tract. Carbohydrate digestion is impaired because of disaccharidase (lactase) deficiency, which is present until 36 weeks of gestational age. Protein is incompletely oxidized to urea and other nitrogen compounds that are excreted in the urine.

Energy Stored

It has been determined that in LBW infants approximately 3.7 Cal must be stored for each gram of weight gained—of which 60–80% is water, 13% is protein, and the rest is fat.[23] The energy expended by a rapidly growing premature infant is expected to exceed that of a slowly growing infant for two reasons: (1) an infant that is fed more expends more calories post-prandially in the digestion process, and (2) more rapid growth requires more energy to synthetize new tissue. In a recent study, the estimated energy cost for 1 g of weight gain for a fast-growing premature infant was 4.5 Cal.[24] In most instances 120 Cal/kg/day provides maintenance for normal infants and allows sufficient calories for growth. Some infants, particularly those who are small for gestational age, have a higher metabolic rate and therefore require more calories. The distribution of caloric expenditure for LBW infants is outlined in Table 4-3.

Fluid Therapy

Maintaining fluid and electrolyte balance is the first nutritional intervention for critically ill neonates in whom regular feedings are not routinely initiated. Simply administering dextrose solutions intravenously to premature infants soon after birth prevents not only dehydration but also the development of hypoglycemia, because hepatic glycogen stores are limited in LBW infants. Basic principles of fluid and electrolyte administration in infants are similar to those established for older children, but the unique body composition of small infants and their impaired neuroendocrine control imposes additional difficulties in fluid management.

Recommended rates of fluid administration for fullterm infants vary from 60–80 cc/kg/day for the first day after birth with progressive increases of 10 cc/kg/day until the 4th postnatal day, when fluid maintenance stabilizes at 100 cc/kg/day. However, for small premature infants the suggested fluid rate for the first few days after birth are significantly higher, ranging from 80–120 cc/kg/day on the first day to 140–180 cc/kg/day on the 3rd, with smaller infants (less than 1 kg) requiring even higher values, 180–200 cc/kg/day.[25] These differences in fluid intake are explained by several characteristics of the very immature infant: its large surface-to-weight ratio; its limited ability to concentrate urine and its large insensible water losses, particularly from the skin–which is thin, has a rich blood supply, a high water content, and an increased permeability.

The nurse caring for sick neonates should be aware of the different factors that increase water losses and thus alter fluid balance. Insensible water losses are significantly increased in infants who are cared for under radiant warmers[26] and in those receiving phototherapy.[27] These losses are magnified when the two therapies are combined.[28] Effective ways of decreasing insensible water losses include covering the infant with a thin plastic film (0.013 mm in diameter), using a plastic shield and providing humidified air (up to 50% humidification) in incubators. If additional fluid is lost through gastrointestinal drainage, vomiting, or diarrheal stools, an equal volume of fluid should be added to the maintenance fluid and the rate of administration should be increased accordingly. Optimal nursing management is achieved by strict monitoring of intake and output and careful measurement of urine specific gravity. In general, a specific gravity greater than 1.010 is compatible with concentrated urine and reflects dehydration. In this circumstance fluid rates should be increased.

ALTERATIONS IN GASTROINTESTINAL TRACT

Gastrointestinal Function

During gestation the fetus receives most nutrients from the mother via the placenta. In addition, the fetus is able to swallow amniotic fluid as early as 16–17 weeks of gestational age. Fetal swallowing at term accounts for nearly half of the total volume of amniotic fluid per day; this intake represents a significant source of protein, as much as 0.6 g/kg/day.

At birth, the newborn infant depends entirely on the gastrointestinal tract for digestion or absorption of nutrients. In the fullterm neonate the enormously complex gastrointestinal mechanisms are well-developed and physiologically efficient. However, the gastrointestinal tract of the premature infant is in an incomplete state of development and is therefore impaired in several physiologic functions.

Gastrointestinal Motility

Despite the demonstrated ability to swallow amniotic fluid in early gestation, sucking mechanisms are not efficient until 33–35 weeks of gestational age. Moreover, the neurological mechanisms that control breathing, sucking, and swallowing are uncoordinated until 35–36 weeks postconception. Three other factors resulting from immaturity that severely limit nutritional intake are an incompetent esophageal sphincter that leads to gastroesophageal reflux; delayed gastric emptying time; and decreased intestinal peristalsis. All of these factors have important clinical implications that should be considered in order to increase the safety of feeding techniques for LBW infants. Impairments in gastrointestinal function of neonates that affect utilization of specific nutrients are incorporated into the section below describing nutritional requirements.

NUTRITIONAL REQUIREMENTS

Protein

Optimal protein intake has not been precisely defined for premature infants. Recommended intakes vary from 2.25 g–5g/kg/day.[29] Protein digestion is initiated in the stomach by pepsin. Pepsin secretion and activity parallel acid secretion in the stomach of neonates and increase rapidly in the first few days of life; pepsin activity then falls to its lowest level between 10–30 days of life. Although lowering proteolytic activity might enhance absorption of antibody protein from colostrum, there is no significant impairment in the proteolytic phase of protein digestion. Ingested proteins are further hydrolyzed by pancreatic trypsin and chymotrypsin. Trypsin response to hormones is decreased in premature infants as compared with that in older children. However, in most newborn infants sufficient trypsin is present for the hydrolysis of protein. Peptides of varying length and solubility, which result from intraluminal hydrolysis of proteins, are then further hydrolyzed by the brush-border peptidases or are directly absorbed. Peptidase activity is present very early in gestation, and levels appear to be unaffected by gestational age.

Weight gain in premature infants fed large amounts of protein (6–9 g/kg/day) does not exceed that in infants fed moderate amounts.[30] In addition, a large intake of protein has been associated with complications such as lethargy and fever,[31] diarrhea,[32] edema,[33] a high BUN level,[34] late metabolic acidosis, and increased mortality.[32] Elevated serum levels of alanine, trysine, proline, and methionine have also been associated with high protein intake.[35] The amino acid composition in milk protein warrants special attention. Cystine, tyrosine, and possibly taurine, which are not required by fullterm infants, are considered to be essential for LBW infants because of the immaturity of their enzymatic metabolic pathways.[36] LBW infants fed protein at whey–casein ratios of 60:40 have lower serum alanine, tyrosine, and ammonia than infants fed casein-predominant formulas with a ratio of 18:82. A high content of cystine is found in breast milk and in formulas with a high whey–casein ratio. In addition, breast milk has a higher taurine level than does any other formula.

When fed at 120 Cal/kg/day, breast milk provides almost 2 g protein/kg/day. Because of its unique amino acid composition, the protein requirement for breast-fed infants is considered to be lower than that for infants fed protein of a whey–casein ratio of 18:82.[37] It has recently been shown that the milk of mothers who deliver prematurely has a higher protein and caloric content than that of mothers who deliver at term.[38] These data suggest the presence of a natural mechanism that regulates the adequacy of human milk for neonates of different gestational ages.

Although soy protein formulas have been used successfully in fullterm infants for specific indications such as sensitivity to cow's milk and diarrheal lactase deficiency, their appropriateness for LBW infants is now being questioned. A recent study done by Shenai et al.[39] showed potential disadvantages of these formulas for LBW infants. These disadvantages included low serum phosphorus and low urinary phosphorus levels, which could lead to the development of phosphorus deficiency rickets. Therefore, the use of these formulas in LBW infants may be undesirable in the absence of specific indications. When LBW infants are fed this type of formula, their protein intake, bone mineralization, and calcium and phosphorus levels must be monitored regularly.

Carbohydrates

Glucose, a carbohydrate metabolite, is an essential nutrient for CNS metabolism. In addition, carbohydrates are an important source of energy and should account for 35–55% of total calories ingested by neonates. Carbohydrates found in human milk and infant formulas are in the form of monosaccharides (glucose), disaccharides (lactose or sucrose), and polysaccharides (starch or glucose polymers); formulas may contain more than one of these substances. Lactose is present in human milk and most infant formulas derived from cow's milk. It has been shown that premature infants are unable to fully digest a load of lactose.[40] Therefore, this sugar should represent only part of the carbohydrate content of formulas prepared for premature infants. Two additional carbohydrates recommended for premature infants are glucose polymers and sucrose.

The addition of sucrose instead of lactose in the preparation of cow's milk formula seems beneficial for LBW infants. A lower incidence of diarrhea and metabolic acidosis has been noted in infants fed these formulas in comparison with those fed formulas containing only lactose.[41] Because lactose is the only carbohydrate present in breast milk, some authorities have questioned the appropriateness of human milk for premature infants. However, a recent study has demonstrated that the concentration of lactose in the milk of a mother who delivers prematurely differs from that of a mother who delivers at term; the milk available to the premature infant has been shown to have lower lactose concentration.[38]

The capacity of the small intestine to hydrolyze disaccharides has been studied by Auricchio et al.[40] Based on these studies, infants born at 36 weeks of gestation can hydrolize only one-third of the quantity of lactose hydrolyzed

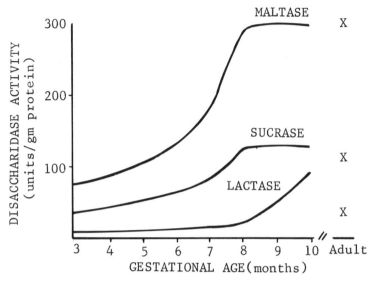

Fig. 4-3.   Source: Fomon, SJ: Gastrointestinal function during infancy. In: Infant Nutrition. 2nd ed. W.B. Saunders Co., 1974, p 104.

by fullterm infants. Other investigators confirmed these findings by detecting a deficiency in intestinal lactase activity. The developmental curve of lactase and other disaccharidases present in the intestinal mucosa are presented in Fig. 4–3.

The intraluminal levels of amylase, the pancreatic enzyme responsible for starch digestion, are very low in neonates. At birth these levels are approximately 10% of adult values, and they remain low for as long as 6 months, after which they increase progressively. No data are available on the development of amylase activity in premature infants, and until such information is known, starches should not be provided as a main source of carbohydrate for premature infants.

Glucose polymers of medium chain length (e.g., corn syrup solids) are common carbohydrate components of infant formulas because they require neither amylase nor lactase for hydrolysis. They appear to be well digested and well tolerated by LBW infants with impaired capacity to digest lactose and sucrose.[42–43] However, except for clinical experience resulting from the use of such formulas, little scientific documentation exists regarding tolerance of glucose polymers in LBW infants. In adults, equicaloric amounts of glucose and glucose polymers are equally well absorbed and metabolized.

Fats

The recommended daily fat intake is 45–50% of the total calories. At least 4% of the total calories should be provided in the form of linoleic acid to meet the requirement for essential fatty acids.

Although fullterm infants absorb up to 90% of ingested lipids, premature infants absorb lipid insufficiently, at rates that vary with gestational age. For instance, premature infants from 32–34 weeks gestational age absorb as little as 65–75% of ingested fat. Since lipids are the nutrients with the highest caloric content, an understanding of the mechanism of fat absorption in LBW infants is of great nutritional importance.

Fats are ingested in the form of triglycerides, molecules resulting from the combination of glycerol with three fatty acid chains. Fat digestion is initiated in the stomach in both adults and premature infants by the lipolysis of the triglycerides. As recently shown by Hamosh,[44] the reaction is mediated by lingual lipase. Further lipolysis occurs in the small intestine, mediated by pancreatic lipase. Pancreatic lipase activity is present as early as the 17th week of gestation and reaches a plateau at 28 weeks, then remains unchanged until term. However, the demonstration of unhydrolized triglyceride in both stools and duodenal aspirates indicates that lipolysis is usually incomplete in premature infants.

The second major step of lipid digestion includes solubilization of the hydrolyzed triglyceride particles through formation of micelles that enter the intestinal mucosa cells. Micelle formation is a process normally carried out by bile salts, which are known to be present in insufficient quantity in premature infants. The bile salt pool in infants born between the 33rd and 37th weeks of gestation is only one-third to one-half of that measured in fullterm infants.[45] Whether this reduction results from either inadequate uptake and synthesis by the liver or from an increased intestinal loss of bile salts is unknown.

The remaining steps of lipid absorption are lipid uptake, triglyceride resynthesis, and chylomicron formation within the intestinal cells. At present, the control mechanisms for these processes are poorly understood in LBW infants. Two aspects that are particularly important in fat digestion in infants are the length of the fatty acid chain and its degree of saturation. Since long chain fatty acids require a high level of bile salt concentration and micelle formation, their absorption is significantly impaired in LBW infants.[46] Saturated lipids often form insoluble calcium soaps in the intestinal lumen, thus increasing steatorrhea and decreasing calcium absorption.

Vegetable oils that contain triglycerides composed of highly unsaturated fatty acids are well-absorbed by the LBW infant and are now used in many formulas for infants. Medium-chain triglycerides (MCT) readily form emulsions that are rapidly hydrolyzed by pancreatic lipase; these compounds are directly absorbed in the portal circulation to the liver independent from micellar formation. For this reason, several commercially available formulas for LBW infants contain MCT as a major lipid source. Fat constitutes 50% of the total calories of human milk. Despite this high content, fat in human milk is well absorbed, because of three major factors: the presence of palmitic acid in position 2 of the triglyceride molecule (as opposed to positions 1 and 3), the high concentration of saturated fatty acids, and the presence of human-milk lipase.

Table 4-4. Infant Formula Nutrient Composition and Recommended Levels for Full Term and LBW Infants (per 100 ml)

Formula	Cal/oz	CHO Source	Protein Source	Fat Source
Minimum level recommended[a]	—	—	—	—
Human milk[b]	22 (20–22)	40% (35–44%) lactose	6% (6–8%) 80% whey 20% casein	54% (35–58%) triglycerides cholesterol phospholipids free fatty acids
Similac Special Care	24	42% 50% lactose 50% corn solids	11% 60% lactose albumin 40% casein	47% 50% MCT oil 30% corn oil 20% coconut oil
Premature formula	24	44% 60% corn syrup solids 40% lactose	12% 60% lactose albumin 40% casein	44% 40% MCT oil 40% corn oil 20% coconut oil
Enfamil without iron	20	41% 100% lactose	9% cow's milk	50% 80% soy oil 20% coconut oil
Similac without iron	20	43% 100% lactose	9% cow's milk	48% 60% coconut oil 40% soy oil
SMA (all Cal levels available only with iron	20	43% 100% lactose	9% 60% lactose albumin 40% casein	48% 33% oleo 27% coconut oil 25% oleic acid 15% soy oil
Similac PM 60/40	20	41% 100% lactose	9% 60% lactose albumin 40% casein	50% 60% coconut oil 40% corn oil
Prosobee	20	40% 100% corn syrup solids	12% soy isolate	48% 80% soy oil 20% coconut oil
Isomil	20	40% 50% corn syrup 50% sucrose	12% soy isolate	48% 60% coconut oil 40% soy oil
Pregestimil	20	54% 85% corn syrup solids 15% modified tapioca starch	11% casein hydrolysate	35% 60% corn oil 40% MCT oil
Portagen	20	46% 75% corn syrup solids 25% sucrose	14% sodium caseinate	40% 85% MCT oil 15% corn oil
Nutramigen	20	52% 72% sucrose 28% modified tapioca starch	13% casein hydrolysate	35% corn oil

[a] Adapted from Committee on Nutrition, American Academy of Pediatrics: Nutritional Needs of Low Birth Weight Infants. Pediatrics, 60(4): 519, 1977

[b] Human milk composition has been shown to vary in mothers depending on gestational age of infants. Table prepared by Sandra Wilson, R.D., Chief Clinical Nutritionist at The Children's Hospital of Philadelphia, Philadelphia, PA

Cal	Protein (g)	Vit D (IU)	Ca (mg)	Folic Acid (mg)	Na (mg/mEq)	Fe (mg)	Ca:P Ratio	% Cal Linoleic	E:PUFA Ratio	mOsm/kg/ H_2O
—	1.2	27	34	2.7	13.4/.6	.1	2:1	4%	1:1	
73 (67–75)	1.0	2.2	34	5	16/.7	.1	2.3:1	8–15%	.7:1	300
80	2.2	118	141	29	34/1.5	.3	2.0:1	10%	3.3:1	300
80	2.4	50	95	20	32/1.4	1.3	2.0:1	10%	1.7:1	300
67	1.5	42	55	11	28/1.2	1.5	1.2:1	20%	.8:1	280
67	1.5	39	50	4.9	24/1.1	tr	1.3:1	12%	1.1:1	290
67	1.5	42	44	5	15/.6	1.3	1.3:1	6%	2:1	300
67	1.5	39	40	5	16/.7	.3	2.0:1	13%	1.0:1	200
67	2.0	42	63	11	29/1.3	1.3	1.3:1	24%	.7:1	200
67	2.0	39	70	9.8	30/1.3	1.2	1.4:1	12%	1.1:1	250
67	1.9	42	63	11	32/1.4	1.3	1.5:1	11%	1.8:1	348
67	2.3	52	63	11	32/1.4	1.3	1.3:1	2.7%	10:1	158
67	2.2	42	63	11	32/1.4	1.3	1.3:1	20%	.7:1	479

Calcium and Phosphorus

Minimum levels of calcium and phosphorus in formulas for LBW infants are 50 mg/100 Cal for calcium and 25 mg/100 Cal for phosphorus. However, some studies have shown that infants fed proprietary formulas containing calcium and phosphorus in concentrations of 2–3 times these recommended values develop better bone texture and wider bone cortexes.[47] Other studies have shown that the use of formulas containing calcium and phosphorus in amounts comparable with the recommended level was not associated with any apparent abnormality of calcium-phorphorus metabolism. This suggests that the current recommendations are not grossly inadequate.[48] Hypocalcemia can be associated with hyperphosphatemia secondary to immature homeostatic control of serum phosphate.[49] Therefore the recommended calcium:phosphorus ratio in formulas for LBW is at least 1.1:1 and ideally is 2:1.[50]

Magnesium

The recommended requirements are based on the human milk content of 6 mg/100 Cal. No cases of magnesium deficiency have been reported in healthy premature infants receiving this recommended amount. All proprietary formulas meet this minimum requirement.

Iron

LBW infants have smaller iron reserves than fullterm infants. When active erythropoiesis occurs between the 1st and 2nd months after birth, the stored iron is rapidly consumed. Therefore, the Committee on Nutrition of the American Academy of Pediatrics recommends that iron supplementation be started by 2 months of age or earlier. Possible disadvantages of early iron supplementation in the first 2 weeks after birth include: (1) an increased susceptibility to vitamin E deficiency and hemolytic anemia, especially when formulas that are used have a high content of polyunsaturated fatty acids,[51] and (2) decreased bacteriostatic activity of human milk proteins (lactoferrin and transferrin) in breast fed infants. Delay in iron supplementation beyond 2 months of age commonly results in the development of iron deficiency anemia in preterm infants.

The Committee on Nutrition recommends that all formulas contain at least the lower level of iron found in human milk (0.15 mg/100 Cal or 1 mg/liter) and that the iron be in bioavailable form. Iron-fortified formulas contain approximately 6–12 mg/liter of this mineral. In spite of the low concentration of iron in human milk, its high bioavailability precludes the need for supplementation in fullterm babies. Iron absorption from human milk is impaired when solid foods are initiated.

Copper

The recommended level of copper for LBW infants is 60 μg/100 Cal, the concentration present in human milk. However, studies have shown that for premature infants a minimum intake of 90 μg/100 Cal is desirable.[52]

Sodium

The minimum recommended level of sodium for fullterm and premature infants is 20 meq/100 Cal. However, hyponatremia has been observed in premature infants fed formulas containing similar concentrations.[53] Therefore, higher levels up to a maximum of 40 meq/100 Cal have been suggested for feeding LBW infants.

Vitamins

In general, proprietary formulas are supplemented with adequate amounts of vitamins that meet the minimum levels recommended for fullterm infants. However, since the milk intake of LBW infants is inadequate, especially in the first 2 weeks after birth, it is important to supply increased amounts of vitamins to these infants. Because there are several reports of deficiency states occurring in premature infants, recommended doses of four vitamins merit attention: vitamin D, folic acid, vitamin B_{12}, and vitamin E. Formulas for premature infants should contain 400 IU of vitamin D/liter, and this requirement may be higher in cases of malabsorption.[54] Folic acid and vitamin B_{12} should be supplemented at daily doses of 50 μg and 1 μg respectively. Vitamin E requirements in LBW infants increase with the amount of polyunsaturated fats in the diet.[55] It is recommended that at least 1.0 IU of vitamin E be present per gram of linoleic acid in the formula. The vitamin E requirement is also increased if the formulas are iron-fortified. The water soluble form of the vitamin is preferable because it is absorbed better. At the time of hospital discharge milk intake is usually sufficient to provide the required vitamins, and further supplementation is no longer necessary.

Human milk, recommended by the Committee on Nutrition of the American Academy of Pediatrics (AAP) as the ideal source of nutrients for fullterm infants, might also be considered a highly desirable nutrient for LBW infants in the near future. As mentioned above, several studies have documented that preterm milk has a higher calorie and protein content and a lower lactose concentration, in addition to its other well-known nutritional, immunologic, and psychologic advantages. The composition of breastmilk and formulas used for premature infants is shown in Table 4-4, along with the AAP's minimum recommended levels.

METHODS OF NUTRITIONAL SUPPORT IN NEONATES

Nutritional support in neonates involves the use of enteral and/or parenteral nutrition. To insure successful and safe delivery of such therapy, every hospital should have a support team composed of physicians, nurses, pharmacists, and nutritionists who provide guidelines for the appropriate application and monitoring of all neonates receiving nutritional therapy.

Enteral Feedings

Techniques for gavage feedings should be standardized in every nursery in the form of a written protocol. Flexibility of these techniques based on the infant's individual needs is the most satisfactory approach.

The following are general guidelines for initiation of enteral feedings:

1. Start with 10–12 Cal/oz formula delivered at 1 cc/kg/hr by constant drip or frequent bolus.
2. Increase the volume by 1–2 ccs every other 8–16 hrs.
3. When one-half the desired volume has been reached, increase the concentration to 20–24 Cal/oz.[56]
4. When full-strength has been reached, increase the volume every 12–24 hrs.
5. Never increase the volume and the concentration simultaneously.
6. Bolus feedings should be administered over at least a 15 min interval.
7. The amount of nutrients received should be meticulously monitored.

The term "residuals" is commonly used to describe the volume of fluid that remains in the stomach from the previous feeding. Its measurement provides important information regarding feeding tolerance and the need for either increasing or decreasing the volume of the next feeding. Residuals should be measured prior to the initiation of each tube feeding. If more than one-half the hourly volume can be aspirated from the stomach, the feeding should be decreased to the previously tolerated volume.

Techniques for Enteral Feeding

Gastric Feeding (Gavage).   Gastric gavage is a method of tube feeding that has been used in nurseries for several decades. This method is recommended for infants with a functional gastrointestinal tract who have an inefficient sucking and/or swallowing mechanism. Indications for gavage feedings include (1) prematurity, (2) neurologic disorders, and (3) respiratory distress caused by either cardiac or pulmonary disease.

The procedure for gavage feeding includes the following:

1. Select a feeding tube with the appropriate caliber: 6–8 French (Fr) for infants weighing more than 2500 g, 5 Fr for infants weighing from 1500–2500 g, and 3.5 Fr for infants of less than 1500 g in weight;
2. Determine the length of the tube to be inserted by measuring the distance from the tip of the nose, to the ear, to the xyphoid process;
3. Insert the tube through either a nostril or the mouth;
4. Check for adequate placement by first injecting 3 cc of air into the tube and listening for the sound of air entry into the stomach by means of a stethoscope and then aspirating the stomach contents;
5. Secure the external part of the tube on the side of the face with a nonirritating tape;

6. Administer feedings through a syringe connected to the feeding tube. An initial gentle "plunge" may be necessary to facilitate flow of the formula. The syringe should remain elevated and the feeding allowed to flow slowly into the stomach by gravity. Feedings should never be "pushed" because acute gastric dilatation may be followed by contraction and cause vomiting.

Gavage feeding tubes can be inserted prior to each feeding or remain indwelling. Both techniques have advantages and disadvantages that need to be considered for individual infants. For instance, in some infants, the intermittent passage of the feeding tube might increase the severity and frequency of apnea by inducing vagal stimulation. On the other hand, indwelling feeding tubes passed by the nose can cause partial upper airway obstruction in neonates known to be obligatory nose breathers. Therefore, caution should be taken when nasal tubes are used for feeding infants with respiratory distress.

In general, indwelling feeding tubes are passed through the nose to increase tolerance and lower the risk of displacement. When passed through the mouth, indwelling tubes enhance mucous production, which necessitates frequent suctioning and retaping of the tube. In addition, tongue movements may also displace part of the tube from the mouth. At the present time, various types of feeding tubes are available. Polyvinyl chloride (PVC) feeding tubes are the most commonly used. Because they become stiff when they remain in the gastrointestinal tract, they should be replaced every 3 days. To avoid trauma to the nasal system, these feeding tubes should be placed in alternate nostrils. Silicone and silastic feeding tubes are also available for neonates and can remain in place for an indefinite length of time. However, because of their softness, guide wires are required to facilitate passage of these tubes.

Transpyloric Feedings (nasojejunal). In 1970, Rhea and Kilby[57] reported the first study on the use of continuous jejunal feedings in sick neonates with tetanus. Since then this method of feeding has become widely used in intensive care nurseries. This method is usually performed according to the modified technique described by Cheek and Staub.[58] The length of the feeding tube to be inserted is determined by using the distance between the eyebrows and the stretched heel as a reference. The tube is then passed through the nose and advanced to either the duodenum or jejunum while the patient is lying on the right side. This position facilitates the tube's passage through the pylorus. To detect adequate placement, the tube is then aspirated and the contents tested. A pH greater than 5 is consistent with placement beyond the pylorus. Confirmation of proper tube positioning is determined by X-ray. It may be necessary to insert the tube more than once before passage through the pylorus occurs. Continuous feedings should always be delivered by means of an infusion pump to provide accurate rates of feedings and minimize the occurrence of the dumping syndrome.

The initial rationale for transpyloric feedings was to diminish the incidence of vomiting and the risk of aspiration. Since then, many studies have reported an increased growth velocity of premature infants fed by the transpyloric route compared with infants fed by the conventional gavage route.[59-61] However, in these studies caloric intake was significantly higher in the infants who received transpyloric feedings; therefore, it remained unclear whether those studies documented a real advantage of the transpyloric route or a less aggressive use of gavage feedings. A recent study on a large number of premature infants in whom transpyloric and gavage feedings were advanced at comparable rates showed no difference in growth, serum protein levels, or feeding-related complications.[62]

Transpyloric feedings have also been associated with high intestinal losses of potassium and fats.[63] These observations suggest that feedings provided by the transpyloric route bypass the stomach where the initial phase of fat digestion by lingual lipase takes place.[64]

The most serious complications of transpyloric feedings have occurred because PVC feeding tubes become rigid with use. These complications, which include gastrointestinal perforation[65] and inability of the stiffened tube to be removed,[66] can be prevented by frequent tube replacement.[67] A better alternative for the administration of pyloric feedings is to use silastic, silicone, or PVC tubes containing non-migrating plasticizers.[67] The potential toxicity from plasticizers leached out of feeding tubes has been documented in vitro and in animal studies but not in humans.[67]

Another complication of transpyloric feedings is called the dumping syndrome, in which the clinical symptoms are diarrhea and abdominal distension. This syndrome can result from rapid delivery of high osmolar feedings (>300 mOsm/liter) into the small intestine. Because transpyloric feedings bypass some of the physiologic and biologic processes that occur in the stomach, this feeding method should not be used on a routine basis. However, transpyloric feedings may be beneficial in situations when the risk of gastric feedings is significant. These include gastroesophageal reflux, severe respiratory distress syndrome, and conditions requiring nasal continuous positive airway pressure.

TOTAL PARENTERAL NUTRITION (TPN)

Total parenteral nutrition is a technique of intravenous feeding designed to meet all the nutritional requirements of patients unable to do so by means of their gastrointestinal (GI) tract. This method of nutrition was first described by Dudrick et al., who demonstrated that both animal and human subjects could sustain normal growth and development while solely nourished by the intravenous route.[68] Despite nutritional benefits of this technique and the significant reduction in surgical mortality of infants born with GI anomalies, this mode of therapy has never been devoid of complications.

Indications

The most common indications for parenteral nutrition in critically ill neonates are (1) congenital anomalies of the GI tract, such as gastroschisis, omphalocele, tracheo-esophageal atresia; (2) acquired GI tract anomalies, such as necrotizing enterocolitis, volvulus, short-bowel syndrome, intestinal perforation; (3) excessive metabolic stress, including RDS, meconium aspiration syndrome, chronic diarrhea, burns; (4) supplemental nutrition to LBW infants with an immature GI tract; (5) inborn errors in metabolism such as glycogen storage disease; and (6) infant botulism.

Composition of TPN Solutions

Table 4-5 details the composition of the TPN solution used at The Children's Hospital of Philadelphia. The volume of nutrients should be based on the fluid requirements of individual infants (80–150 cc/kg/day). Caloric content of the infused solutions should also match caloric requirements for neonates, which vary from 100–120 Cal/kg/day (see caloric and fluid requirement in section above).

Amino acids. Proteins in TPN solutions are provided as either protein hydrolysates or crystalline amino-acid solutions. Protein hydrolysates—the first source of protein manufactured for intravenous use—consist of approximately 55% amino acids and 45% dipeptides and tripeptides. Use of these earlier preparations resulted in metabolic acidosis because of their high content of chloride salts. More recently, crystalline and amino-acid solutions have become available for clinical use. These solutions are derived from proteins of high biologic value such as egg albumin, and their use is associated with significantly fewer metabolic complications.

Intravenous protein and nitrogen requirements in infants are estimated to vary from 2–3 g/kg/day and 0.315 g/kg respectively. The catabolism of each gram of protein administered results in approximately 4 Cal. However, infused

Table 4-5. The Children's Hospital of Philadelphia
Parenteral Nutrition Solution

	Per 500 ml of solution
Aminosyn 10%	2.0–2.5 g/kg/day
Dextrose	10–50%
Sodium Cl°°	20–40 mEq
Potassium Cl°°	10–20 mEq
Ca gluconate	5 mEq
Magnesium	2 mEq
Phosphate, potassium	7 mEq
Zinc	1500 μg
Copper	150 μg
Chromium	1 μg
Manganese	50 μg
Folic acid	200 μg
Vitamin B_{12}	2.5 μg
MVI concentrate	2.5 ml
Berrocca 'C'	.3 ml
Heparin	500 units

°° should be adjusted according to daily electrolytes; Vitamin K, 1 mg given IM once a week proteins should not be counted as a source of "utilizable energy" but rather as a source of nitrogen for protein synthesis and formation of new tissue necessary for growth. When protein is provided intravenously, it is necessary to maintain a ratio of 1 g of nitrogen (which is contained in 6.25 g of protein) to at least 150–250 nonprotein Cal to prevent protein catabolism.

Carbohydrates.   Glucose, the most common of all sugars, is commercially available as dextrose solution (so called because of the dextrorotatory property of the glucose molecule). The neonate—especially the premature infant—has a limited ability to tolerate glucose. However, glucose tolerance improves steadily after the first few postnatal days both because an increased amount of insulin is secreted and because organ sensitivity to insulin increases.[69] The use of sugars such as galactose and fructose is associated with delayed serum clearance rates, high urinary excretory levels, and moderate to severe lactic acidosis. Their use in the neonate offers no clinical advantage over the use of glucose.

TPN solutions are usually initiated with a 10% concentration of dextrose. However, when high rates of infusates (greater than 150 cc/kg/day) are delivered, the total glucose load may not be tolerated and hyperglycemia will result. This is particularly likely in premature infants weighing less than 1500 g. Under these circumstances glucose concentrations should be reduced. After the 2nd week of postnatal life most neonates tolerate higher dextrose concentrations if increments are made slowly and progressively.

Dextrose solutions of 20–50% concentration can be administered if a central line for delivery of these high osmolar solutions is available. The combination of dextrose and amino acids is preferred to either amino acids alone or amino acids plus fat in conditions of high metabolic stress such as trauma, the immediate postoperative period, and critical illness.[70] Each gram of infused dextrose provides approximately 3.4 Cal.

Fats.   Along with amino acids and dextrose, fats are an essential component of a TPN regimen. There are at least three advantages of using fats intravenously. They are a source of essential fatty acids; their caloric density is high; and they have a low osmolality suitable for peripheral vein use. At least 4% of total calories should be provided as linoleic acid to prevent essential fatty acid deficiency. Intravenous administration of fats is commonly initiated at daily doses of 1 g/kg and progressively advanced to maximal daily doses of 3 g/kg, provided that calories from fat do not exceed 50% of the total calories received.

Fats for intravenous administration are presently manufactured as either 10% or 20% emulsions that should be administered separately from other TPN components to preserve the stability of the emulsion.

Neonates are given an initial test dose of 1 ml fat intravenously over 15 min. If no adverse effects (e.g., hypotension, vomiting, fever) occur, the infusion of lipids is then started at a rate of 1 g/kg/day. Shennan et al.[71] have reported that in premature infants older than 33 weeks gestational age, 0.3 g/kg/hr is the safe maximal dose of lipids with adequate serum clearance. Premature infants less than 33 weeks of gestation should not receive more than

0.16 g/kg/hr. To prevent hyperlipemia, it is strongly recommended that a baseline measurement of free fatty acids, triglycerides, and cholesterol be done in all neonates who receive intravenous fats. Serial measurements should be done whenever the dose of fat is increased and then weekly thereafter. A practical but unreliable indicator of hyperlipemia is "cloudy serum," which can be observed after centrifugation of blood samples.

Potential complicatons that might result from the use of intravenous fats in LBW infants include (1) deposition of lipid particles in the pulmonary microcirculation impairing oxygenation, especially in the first postnatal week;[72] (2) competition of resultant free fatty acids with bilirubin for albumin-binding sites;[73] and (3) decreased production of complement (C2) and impaired phagocytosis of white cells.[74] Therefore, caution should be applied when using intravenous fats in patients with severe respiratory distress, high levels of jaundice, and susceptibility to bacterial infections. Under these circumstances, fat infusion should be temporarily decreased or discontinued. However, minimum weekly doses of 1 g/kg/day should be provided, because a fat-free TPN regimen in neonates quickly leads to the development of essential-fatty-acid deficiency. This deficiency is clinically expressed by dermatitis, hemolytic anemia, impaired wound healing, increased susceptibility to bacterial infection, and growth retardation. Commercially available intravenous fat emulsions are mainly composed of long-chain fatty acids of high caloric value. Each gram of the 10% emulsion provides 11 Cal.

Table 4-6. Recommended Dietary Allowances (RDA) for Vitamins and Suggested Formulations for Intravenous and Intramuscular Use[a]

Vitamins	RDA				Suggested formulations	
	Range infants (/kg body wt 0.0–0.5 and 0.5–1.0 yr)	Mean infant	Range children under 11 years	AAP[b] minimum/100 Cal orally	Multivitamin[c] for intravenous use for under 11 yrs	Water-soluble vitamins for intra muscular use
A (retinol), IU	233–222	227.0	2,000–3,300	250.0	2,300[d]	
D, IU	66–44	55.0	400	40.0	400.0[e]	
E (α tocopherol), IU	0.66–0.55	0.6	7–10	0.3	7.0	
K₁ (phylloquinone), mg					0.2	
Ascorbic acid, mg	6–4	5.0	40	8.0	80.0	80.0
Folacin, μg	8–6	7.0	100–300	4.0	140.0	140.0
Niacin, mg	0.9–0.8	0.85	9–16	0.25	17.0	17.0
Riboflavin, mg	0.07	0.07	0.8–1.2	0.06	1.4	1.4
Thiamin, mg	0.055–0.05	0.053	0.7–1.2	0.025	1.2	1.2
B₆ (pyridoxine), mg	0.05–0.04	0.045	0.6–1.2	0.035	1.0	1.0
B₁₂ (cyanocobalamin), μg	0.04–0.03	0.035	1–2	0.15	1.0	1.0
Pantothenic acid, mg				0.3	5.0[f]	5.0
Biotin, μg					20.0[f]	20.0

[a] Adapted from Tables 1, 2, and 4, Guidelines for Multivitamin Preparations for Parenteral Use, AMA, 1975; J Parent. Ent. Nutr, 3:258–261, 1979. Reprinted with the permission of the American Medical Association.

[b] American Academy of Pediatrics.[2]

[c] May be provided in in appropriate salt or ester form in equivalent potency.

[d] 700 μg of retinol.

[e] As ergocalciferol or cholecalciferol.

[f] RDA not established; amount = 20 × 100 kcal human milk.

Table 4-7. Suggested Daily Intravenous Intake of Minerals and Essential Trace Elements in Children[a]

	kg/day
Sodium (mEq)[b]	3–5
Potassium (mEq)[b]	1–2
Magnesium (mEq)[b]	0.3–0.5
Calcium (mg)	20–40
Phosphorus (mg)	20–40
Iron (mg)	1.0[c]
Zinc (μg)[d]	300[e]
	100[f]
Copper (μg)	20
Chromium (μg)	0.14–0.2
Manganese (μg)	2–10
Fluoride (mg)[g]	0.001
Iodide (μg)[h]	3–5

[a] Adapted from Guidelines for Essential Trace Element Preparations for Parenteral Use, AMA, 241:2051–2054 1979; J Parent Ent Nutr, 3:263–266 1979 and Goodhart R, Shils M: Modern Nutrition in Health and Disease, 6th edn, Philadelphia, Lea & Febiger, 1980. © The American Society of Parenteral and Enteral Nutrition.

[b] For patients without significant cardiovascular renal dysfunction or intestinal or renal losses. The upper range is suggested for those with rapid growth rate.

[c] May be given periodically as indicated for correcting deficiency.

[d] Limited data available for infants weighing less than 1500 g. Their requirements may be higher because of low body reserves and rapid growth.

[e] Premature infant weight 1500 g–3 kg. Thereafter, recommendations for fullterm infants apply.

[f] Fullterm infants and children up to 5 years. Thereafter, recommendations for adults apply (2.5–4.0 mg).

[g] Human requirements probable but not definite; range very uncertain.

[h] Human requirements definite-range uncertain.

Minerals and Vitamins

Tables 4-6 and 4-7 present the AAP and RDA requirements for vitamins and minerals in infancy.

Modes of Therapy

Peripheral Vein. Parenteral nutrition by the peripheral vein route is indicated for infants in whom the need for nutritional support is expected to be of relatively short duration, usually less than 2 weeks.

In general, peripheral route solutions used in neonates are provided at maximal dextrose concentrations of 10% in order to avoid skin sloughing. Therefore, caloric restriction is a major limitation of peripheral-vein parenteral nutrition, and the use of intravenous fats is necessary to achieve adequate caloric intake. Lipids should be administered at maximum rates of 3g/kg/day. At maintenance fluid rates, peripheral route solutions maximally provide 80–90 Cal/day, which prevents weight loss but does not promote adequate growth.

Peripheral-vein alimentation is commonly used to supplement feedings for LBW infants. In 1974, Cashore et al.[75] reported that premature infants could reach growth velocities comparable with intrauterine rates if their feedings were routinely supplemented with intravenous dextrose, amino acids, and fat emulsions. When feedings for LBW infants are supplemented, the volume and caloric density of the provided nutrients should be closely monitored.

Solutions for intravenous nutrition should be continued until the enteral feedings have advanced to 20–24 Cal/oz and provide at least 75% of the total calories. During this weaning process a careful plan for modifying the volumes of the nutrients received by both parenteral and enteral routes is important to insure adequate caloric intake.

A major nursing responsibility includes close observation of the rate of the solutions infused by a volumetric pump. In addition, the peripheral vein site should be monitored hourly for signs of fluid infiltration or phlebitis. It is mandatory that peripheral vein catheters be changed every 72 hrs to preserve venous accessibility; preferably, this should be done by a nurse experienced in intravenous insertion.

Central Vein.   Central vein catheters are indicated for the delivery of TPN solutions under the following conditions: (1) when the duration of nutritional therapy is expected to exceed 2 weeks, (2) when accessibility to peripheral veins is difficult; (3) in fluid-restricted neonates who require TPN, and (4) when daily intravenous caloric requirements exceed 100 Cal/kg.

The venous catheter tip is placed at the junction of the superior vena cava and the right atrium, a region where high blood flow allows rapid dilution of the hypertonic infusates, thus preventing venous inflammation and thrombosis. The catheters used can be made of PVC or silastic. The use of silastic catheters has been associated with a lower risk of venous thrombosis and fibrin depostion around the catheter tip.

Techniques for catheter placement include the method described by Dudrick et al.[68] in which the superior vena cava is cannulated from the jugular vein and the catheter is then tunneled subcutaneously from the vein entry point to an exit site located on the scalp or anterior chest. This tunneled exit site offers several advantages: it facilitates proper cleaning, decreases the possibility of accidental removal of the catheter, minimizes the risk of systemic infection, and allows freedom of movement. This method requires that the infant be transferred to the operating room so that general anesthesia can be used and adequate asepsis can be assured.

More recently, a technique for percutaneous catheterization of the subclavian vein has been described and successfully used at The Children's Hospital of Philadelphia to deliver parenteral nutrition solutions in infants. This method requires that the infant be immobilized and placed in the Trendelenburg position.

Catheter Care

Meticulous catheter care must be provided to all infants with central venous lines to minimize the chance of infection introduced by pathogens. Dressings should be changed every other day or more often in patients with a tracheostomy or excessive drooling. In addition to strict adherence to aseptic technique, the steps of the procedure are as follows:

1. Wear a mask to avoid contaminating the catheter site.
2. Position the infant with his head turned toward the side opposite to that of the catheter.
3. Open the dressing tray.
4. Remove the old dressing and place it in a plastic bag.
5. Check the insertion site for signs of infection, intact sutures, signs of infiltration, and skin irritation.
6. Put on sterile gloves.
7. Wipe the insertion site and outer periphery with acetone-alcohol to defat the skin, making sure to use friction when wiping. Avoid contact between a catheter that is made of PVC and the swab, because the acetone-alcohol makes the PVC dry and brittle.
8. Cleanse the exit site and outer periphery with povidone-iodine solution, again using a lot of friction.
9. Remove the povidone-iodine solution with a sterile gauze pad.
10. Apply povidone-iodine ointment to the exit site and the sutures.
11. Apply a sterile 2″ × 2″ gauze dressing over the exit site.
12. Cover the gauze with a non-irritating tape, one that does not alter the normal flora of the skin.
13. Secure the catheter with tape so that the dressing is occlusive.
14. Label the dressing with the date and your initials.
15. Chart the dressing change, condition of the site, and any other pertinent information.

Monitoring

Table 4-8 lists the suggested biochemical parameters that should be followed in all children who are receiving TPN in order that complications can be prevented from occurring.

Metabolic Complications of Parenteral Nutrition

Hyperglycemia. Unless it is precipitated by infection, hyperglycemia is observed mainly in LBW premature infants. In the absence of infection, a temporary decrease in the rate of infusion or in the dextrose concentration of the solution usually returns the serum-glucose level to normal. Once normoglycemia is achieved for at least 24 hrs, the dextrose concentration can then be gradually increased to its original strength. If these adjustments fail to lower the serum glucose level, the use of exogenous insulin may be necessary.

Hypoglycemia. Rebound hypoglycemia occasionally occurs following abrupt cessation of TPN with a hypertonic dextrose solution. This reaction, which is triggered by the high levels of circulating insulin that are produced

Table 4-8. Parenteral Nutrition Monitoring Protocol from The Children's Hospital of Philadelphia Nutrition Support Service

Blood

Glucose Electrolytes	daily until stable
BUN Ca, PO_4, Mg Alk Phos, SGOT, SGPT, Bilirubin, T/D Creatinine Total protein, albumin CBC with differential	weekly
Serum lipemia Triglycerides, cholesterol Metabolic screen	as indicated
Zinc, copper	monthly (1st of each month)
Other trace elements	as indicated
Dextrostix (infants only)	when TPN is abruptly discontinued or when spilling +2 glucose in urine

Urine

Glucose Protein Ketone Specific gravity pH	every 4 hr until stable, then every 8 hr
Metabolic screen	as indicated

General

Vital signs	every 4 hrs
Weight Strict intake and output Caloric intake	daily
Length Head circumference	weekly (every Mon)

in response to the elevated dextrose load of the infusate, may be avoided by gradually decreasing both the concentration of the dextrose load and the rate of infusion. The process usually requires approximately 2 days.

Glycosuria.   The appearance of glucose in the urine indicates that serum glucose levels are exceeding the renal threshold. Premature infants have a lower renal threshold for glucose than fullterm infants. Decreasing the rate of infusion or the dextrose concentration usually returns the serum glucose value to normal and promptly improves glycosuria unless another problem such as infection is present.

Osmotic Diuresis.   This complication occasionally occurs secondary to significant glycosuria when a 25% dextrose solution is used. Premature infants with underdeveloped renal tubular function are more susceptible to this complication. Osmotic diuresis is rarely a problem in infants treated with peripheral hyperalimentation, because peripheral solutions are, by necessity, of lower dextrose concentration.

Essential Fatty Acid Deficiency.   The ramifications of a deficiency in essential fatty acids can be extensive. Fortunately, the incidence of this complication has been substantially reduced by the routine administration of commercial intravenous fat emulsions. Clinical signs of essential fatty acid deficiency can occur as early as 1–3 weeks after initiation of nutritional therapy if fat infusions are not provided.

Some of the more serious effects of this disorder are growth retardation, inhibition of prostaglandin synthesis, and impairment of the cholesterol-transport mechanism. Other effects include a generalized skin rash and changes in the mitochondrial membranes of hepatic cells. Probably the most typical abnormality associated with essential fatty acid deficiency is an increase in the serum concentrations of 5,8,11-eicosatrienoic acid.

Essential fatty acid deficiency can be prevented by providing 4% of the infant's daily caloric requirement in the form of linoleic acid, the essential fatty acid that is not produced by the body. This can be accomplished by one of two methods: intravenous infusion of a fat emulsion or daily topical application of sunflower seed oil to the chest. Most patients treated intravenously maintain normal serum cholesterol and triglyceride levels; however, if the period of parenteral nutrition exceeds 1 month, the patient may exhibit mild elevations in the levels of both these lipids. The serum triglyceride level may increase to 300–350 mg% (normal: 150–250 mg%) and the serum cholesterol level to 150–250 mg% (normal: 100–150 mg%). Both values return to normal once the infusion of fat is discontinued.

Vitamin Deficiency.   A multivitamin preparation suitable for intravenous use (Multivitamin) is used to supply most vitamins. However, vitamin B_{12}, folic acid, and biotin are not included in this preparation and must be added separately to TPN solutions (see Table 4-6 for dosages). Vitamin K also is not present in commercial vitamin products and must be administered intramuscularly in 1-mg weekly doses until gastrointestinal feedings are initiated.

Hypocalcemia, Hypercalcemia, Hypophosphatemia, and Hyperphosphatemia.   Although these complications have occurred in patients fed solely by vein, they have not been observed in most of the patients treated with the solutions described in this chapter. The quantities of calcium and phosphorus in these solutions are sufficient to avoid these problems in most infants. With close monitoring of the serum calcium and phosphorus values, such complications are easily detected and corrected.

Cholestatic Jaundice.   Cholestasis seems to be the most common metabolic complication in LBW infants. Although its etiology is unknown, it occurs with greater frequency in less mature infants, especially in association with bacterial infections and prolonged use of TPN solutions.[76] This complication usually resolves as gastrointestinal feedings are initiated and TPN solutions are progressively discontinued. However, chronic liver disease with resultant cirrhosis has been reported in patients dependent on TPN for extended periods of time.[77]

Infectious Complications. Sepsis continues to be the major complication of central parenteral nutrition in patients of all ages, particularly in infants. Organisms may enter the blood stream via the catheter and the parenteral solution. The venous catheter, as a foreign body, may be a focus for the growth of organisms, thus causing bacteremia and possibly infections at sites quite distant from the catheter. Strict aseptic technique and appropriate nursing care of the catheter site, as outlined above helps significantly to reduce the incidence of this complication. In addition, restriction of the use of the central catheter for drawing blood or administering medications helps to prevent bacterial contamination. The incidence of infection also seems to be related to the length of time the catheter has been in place.[76,77]

Sepsis can also result from bacterial contamination of nutritional solutions. All TPN solutions should be prepared by an experienced pharmacist using aseptic technique under a laminar air flow hood. Quality control measures include (1) obtaining surveillance cultures from 1 of every 10 TPN bottles prepared, (2) keeping prepared solutions refrigerated and using them within 48 hrs after preparation, (3) discouraging introduction of additives to TPN solutions by nurses in the hospital wards, and (4) changing the soluset delivery system and solution daily.

The development of sepsis almost always necessitates removing the central line unless the patient has an identifiable source of infection unrelated to that line. Under the latter circumstances antimicrobial treatment is initiated without removal of the central line. However, blood cultures—including one of a sample obtained through the central line are indicated. Moreover, the TPN bottle that is used should always be cultured as part of patient management.

CONCLUSIONS

Nutritional support by either the enteral or the parenteral route can be delivered safely to critically ill neonates. Significant advances in nutrition are occurring rapidly. Special nutrition solutions are now available for infants in renal or hepatic failure. Infant formulas are being redesigned to better meet the needs of the LBW infants. Therefore, to ensure optimal therapy, it is imperative that a dedicated team of physicians, nurses, pharmacists, and nutritionists experienced in the field of nutrition support monitor all infants who require special nutritional therapies. Neonatal critical care nurses can greatly contribute to this goal by continuing to expand their knowledge of the physiologic principles of infant metabolism and the methods for recognizing nutritional deficit.

REFERENCES

1. Wegman ME: Newborn infant mortality: Annual summary of vital statistics—1974. Pediatrics 56:960, 1975
2. Stoch MB, Smythe PM: Does undernutrition during infancy inhibit brain growth and subsequent intellectual development? Arch Dis Child 38:546, 1963
3. Winick M, Noble A: Cellular response in rats during malnutrition at various ages. J Nutr 89:300, 1966
4. Winick M, Rosso P: Head circumference and cellular growth of the brain in normal and marasmic children. J Pediatr 74:774, 1969
5. Winick M: Cellular growth in intrauterine malnutrition. Pediatr Clin North Am 17:69, 1970
6. Christensen RD, Rothstein G: Exhaustion of mature marrow neutrophils in neonates with sepsis. J Pediatr 96:316, 1980
7. Wright WC Jr, Ank BJ, Herbst J, et al.: Decreased bacteriocidal activity of leukocytes of stressed newborn infants. Pediatrics 56:579, 1975
8. Stoerner JW, Pickering LK, Adcock EW III, et al.: Polymorphonuclear leukocyte function in newborn infants. J Pediatr 93:862, 1978
9. Weston WL, Carson BS, Barkin RM, et al.: Monocyte-macrophage function in the newborn. Am J Dis Child 131:1241, 1977
10. Schuit KE, DeBiasio R: Kinetics of phagocyte response to group B streptococcal infections in newborn rats. Infect Immun 28:310, 1980
11. McCracken GH Jr, Eichenwald HF: Leukocyte function and the development of opsonic and complement activity in the neonate. Am J Dis Child 121:120, 1971
12. Lubchenco LO: Long term followup studies of prematurely born infants. I. Relationship of handicaps to nursery routines. J Pediatr 30:501, 1972
13. Mullen JL, Buzby GP, Mathews DC, et al.: Reduction of operative morbidity and mortality by combined pre and post-operative nutritional support. Br J Surg 66:893, 1979
14. Driver AG, McAlevy MT, Burgher LW: Nutritional support of patients with respiratory failure. Nutr Suppl Serv 1:26, 1981
15. Committee on Nutrition, American Academy of Pediatrics: Nutritional needs of low birthweight infants. Pediatrics 60:519, 1977
16. Tanner JM: Physical growth and development. In: Textbook of Pediatrics. eds. Forfar JO and Arneil GC. London, Churchill Livingstone, 1973
17. Bland RD: Cord blood total protein level as a screening aid for the idiopathic respiratory distress syndrome. N Engl J Med 287:9, 1972
18. Pereira GR, Lemons JA: A controlled study of transpyloric and intermittent gavage feeding in the small preterm infant. Pediatrics 67:68, 1981
19. Oganshima SO, Hussain MA: Plasma thyroxine binding pre-albumin as an index of protein energy malnutrition in Nigerian children. Am J Clin Nutr 33:794, 1980
20. Inglebleek Y, Van Der Schriek HG, DeNayer P, et al.: The role of retinol binding protein in protein caloric malnutrition. Metabolism 24:633, 1975
21. Narasinga Rao BS, Nagabhushan VS: Urinary excretion of 3-methylhistidine in children suffering from protein–calorie malnutrition. Life Sci 12:205, 1973
22. Ballard FJ, Tomas LM, Pope PG: Muscle protein degradation in premature infants. Clin Sci 57:535, 1979
23. Gordon H, Levine S, Deamer W, et al.: Respiratory metabolism in infancy and childhood. XXII. Daily energy requirements of premature infants. Am J Dis Child 59:1185, 1940

24. Sinclair J, Whyte RK, Haslam R, et al.: Energy balance during extrauterine growth of the very low birthweight infant. Proceedings of the 79th Ross Conference on Pediatric Research, 1979, pp 15
25. Fanaroff AA, Hack M: Meeting nutritional needs of infants less than 1500 grams: implications, risks and benefits. Proceedings of the 79th Ross Conference on Pediatric Research, 1979, p 3
26. Williams PR, Oh W: Effect of radiant warmer on insensible water loss in newborn infants. Am J Dis Child 128:511, 1974
27. Oh W, Karecki H: Phototherapy and insensible water loss in the newborn infant. Am J Dis Child 124:230, 1972
28. Engle WD, Baumgart S, Schwartz JG, et al.: Insensible water loss in the critically ill neonate—combined effect of radiant warmer power and phototherapy. Am J Dis Child 135:516, 1981
29. Cox WM Jr, Filer LJ Jr: Protein intake for low birth weight infants. J Pediatr 74:1016, 1969
30. Davidson M, Levine SZ, Bauer CH, et al.: Feeding studies in low birth weight infants. I. Relationships of dietary protein, fat, and electrolytes to rates of weight gain, clinical courses and serum chemical concentrations. J Pediatr 70:965, 1967
31. Goldman HI, Freudenthal R, Holland B, et al.: Clinical effects of two different levels of protein intake on low birth weight infants. J Pediatr 74:881, 1969
32. Omans WB, Barness LA, Rose CS, Gyorgy P: Prolonged feeding studies in premature infants. J Pediatr 59:951, 1961
33. Snyderman SE, Boyer A, Kogut MD, Holt LE Jr: The protein requirement of the premature infant. I. The effects of protein intake on the retention of nitrogen. J Pediatr 74:872, 1969
34. Nichols MM, Danford BH: Feeding premature infants: a comparison of effects of weight gain, blood and urine of two formulas with varying protein and ash composition. South Med J 59:1420, 1966
35. Levine SZ, Gordon HH, Marples E: A defect in the metabolism of tyrosine and phenylalanine in premature infants. II. Spontaneous occurrence and eradication by vitamin C. J Clin Invest 20:209, 1941
36. Snyderman SE, Holt LE Jr, Norton PM, Phansalkar SV: Protein requirement of the premature infant. II. Influence of protein intake on free amino acid content of plasma and red blood cells. Am J Clin Nutr 23:890, 1970
37. Committee on Nutrition, American Academy of Pediatrics: Nutritional needs of low birth weight infants. In: Pediatric Nutrition Handbook. ed. Committee on Nutrition. Evanston, IL, 1979 pp 92–118
38. Anderson GH, Atkinson SA, Bryan MH: Energy and micronutrient content of human milk during early lactation from mothers giving birth prematurely and at term. Am J Clin Nutr 34:258, 1981
39. Shenai JP, Jhaveri BM, Reynolds JW, et al.: Nutritional balance studies in very low birth weight infants. The role of soy formula. Pediatrics 67:631, 1981
40. Auricchio S, Rubino A, Mursett G.: Intestinal glycosidase activities in the human embryo, fetus and newborn. Pediatrics 35:944, 1965
41. Fosbrooke AS, Wharton BA: "Added lactose" and "added sucrose" cow's milk formula in nutrition for low birth weight babies. Arch Dis Child 50:409, 1975
42. Cicco R, Holzman I, Brown DR, et al.: Glucose polymer tolerance in premature infants. Pediatrics 67:498, 1981
43. Boellner SE, Beard AG, Panos TC: Impairment of intestinal hydrolysis of lactose in newborn infants. Pediatrics 36:542, 1965

44. Hamosh M: A review on fat digestion in the newborn. Role of lingual lipase and pre-jejunal digestion. Pediatr Res, 13:615, 1979
45. Watkins JB, Szezepanik P, Gould JB, et al.: Bile salt metabolism in the human premature infant. Gastroenterology 69:706, 1975
46. Watkins JB: Infant nutrition and the development of gastrointestinal function. In: Pediatric Nutrition Handbook. ed. Committee on Nutrition, American Academy of Pediatrics, Evanston, IL, 1979 pp 58–69
47. Day GM, Chance GW, Radde IC, et al.: Growth and minimal metabolism in very low birth weight infants. II. Effects of calcium supplementation on growth and divalent cations. Pediatr Res 9:568 1975
48. Barness LA, Omans WB, Rose CS, et al.: Progress of premature infants fed a formula containing demineralized whey. Pediatrics 32:52, 1963
49. Oppe TE, Redstone D: Calcium and phosphorus levels in healthy newborn infants given various types of milk. Lancet 1:1045, 1968
50. Committee on Nutrition: Commentary on breastfeeding and infant formulas including proposed standards for formulas. Pediatrics 57:278, 1976
51. Williams ML, Shott RJ, O'Neal PL, Oski FA: Role of dietary iron and fat on vitamin E deficiency anemia of infancy. N Engl J Med 292:887, 1975
52. Cordano A: The role played by copper in the physiopathology and nutrition of the infant and child. Ann Nestle 33:5, 1974
53. Honour JW, Shackleton CHL, Valman HB: Sodium homeostasis in premature infants. Lancet 2:1147, 1974
54. Lewin PK, Reid M, Reilly BJ, et al.: Iatrogenic rickets in low birth weight infants. J Pediatr 78:207, 1971
55. Dallman PR: Iron, vitamin E, and folate in the preterm infant. J Pediatr 85:742, 1974
56. Kaminski MV: Enteral hyperalimentation. Surg Gyn Obstr 143:13, 1976
57. Rhea JW, Kilby JO: A nasojejunal tube for infant feeding. Pediatrics 46:36, 1970
58. Cheeck JA Jr, Staub GF: Nasojejunal alimentation for premature and full-term newborn infants. J Pediatr 82:955, 1973
59. Wells DH, Zachman RD: Nasojejunal feeding in low birth weight infants. J Pediatr 87:277, 1975
60. Wolfsdorf J, Makarawa S, et al: Transpyloric feeding in small preterm infants. Arch Dis Child, 50:723, 1975
61. VanCaille M, Powell GK: Nasoduodenal vs. nasogastric feeding in the very low birth weight infant. Pediatrics, 56:1065, 1975
62. Pereira GR, Lemons JA: A comparative study between transpyloric and gavage feeding in preterm infants. Pediatr Res 10:358, 1976
63. Roy RN, Pollmitz RP, Hamilton JR, et al.: Impaired alimentation of nasojejunal feedings in healthy low birth weight newborn infants. J Pediatr 90:431, 1977
64. Hamosh M: A review on fat digestion in the newborn: role of lingual lipase and prejejunal digestion. Pediatr Res 13:615, 1979
65. Boros SJ, Reynolds JW: Duodenal perforation. A complication of neonatal naso-jejunal feedings. J Pediatr 85:107, 1974
66. Hayhurst EG, Wyman M: Morbidity associated with prolonged use of polyvinyl feeding tubes. Am J Dis Child 129:72, 1975
67. Pereira GR, Herold R, Ziegler M, et al.: Increased safety of polyvinylchloride (PVC) tubes used for enteral feedings in newborn infants. J Parent Ent Nutr 4:601, 1982

68. Dudrick SJ, Wilmore DW, Vars HM, et al.: Long term total parenteral nutrition with growth, development and positive nitrogen balance. Surgery 64:134, 1968
69. Pollack A, Cowett RM, Schwartz R, et al.: Glucose disposal in low birth weight infants during steady state hyperglycemia: effects of exogenous insulin administration. Pediatrics 61:546, 1978
70. Long JM: Effect of energy source on nitrogen. In: Clinical Nutrition Update—Amino acids. eds. Greene HL, Holiday MA, Munro HN. Chicago, IL, American Medical Assoc, 1977 pp 79–81
71. Shennan AT, Bryan MH, Angel A: The effect of gestational age on Intralipid tolerance in newborn infants. J Pediatr, 91:134, 1977
72. Pereira GR, Fox WW, Stanely CA, et al.: Decreased oxygenation and hyperlipemia during intravenous fat infusion in preterm infants. Pediatrics 66:26, 1980
73. Andrew G, Chan G, Schiff D: Lipid metabolism in the neonate. II. The effect of Intralipid on bilirubin binding in vitro and in vivo. J Pediatr 88:279, 1976
74. Fisher GW, Hunter KW, Wilson SR, et al.: Inhibitory effect of Intralipid on reticuloendothelial function and neutrophil bacteriocidal activity. Pediatr Res 13:494, 1979
75. Cashore WJ, Sedaghatian MR, Usher RN: Nutritional supplements with intravenously administered lipids, protein hydrolysate and glucose in small premature infants. Pediatrics 56: 8, 1975
76. Pereira GR, Ziegler M, Roth K, et al.: Clinical factors associated with hyperalimentation induced cholestasis in neonates. J Parent Ent Nutr 3:510, 1979
77. Pereira GR, Sherman M, DiGiacomo J, et al.: Increased incidence and severity of hyperalimentation induced cholestasis in premature infants. Am J Dis Child 135:842, 1981

5 | Current Trends and Conflicts in Perinatal Research

Alan R. Spitzer
Kit Stahler-Miller

Few areas of modern medicine have witnessed as many significant changes and advances during the past two decades as the field of neonatology. As recently as the early 1960s no true newborn intensive care units (NICUs) existed in the United States. The country was made painfully aware of this shortcoming when the son of President John F. Kennedy was born prematurely and developed hyaline membrane disease. After a rapidly deteriorating course the baby died when treatment with hyperbaric oxygen failed. Today that child's chances for survival, in view of his size and gestational age, would be excellent. Immediately after this event, possibly stimulated by the general awareness that neonatal care lagged substantially behind other branches of medicine, the modern era of neonatology began.

The first NICUs appeared in the mid-1960s, and their success soon became apparent. Survival rates for numerous illnesses steadily improved, often very dramatically. As the wealth of conventional and newly developed technology was applied to the care of newborns it quickly became clear that increasing numbers of smaller, more critically ill infants would survive. Of even more importance, follow-up data showed that the quality of life for these survivors significantly outstripped initial expectations. However, problems, such as the epidemic of blindness that resulted from retrolental fibroplasia (RLF) induced by overexposure to inspired oxygen, made people aware of the need to correlate symptom-directed therapy with ultimate total outcome. In addition, the continual impetus to save immature babies made physicians and nurses aware of the large gaps in knowledge that existed regarding the physiology and development of the premature infant. Thus, the era of perinatal research was ushered in.

THE MODERN ERA OF PERINATAL RESEARCH

The history of perinatal research antedates the improvements in the clinical care of the sick neonate that began in the 1960s. The first significant explorations into newborn physiology occurred with the publication of Sir Joseph Barcroft's *Researches on Prenatal Life*[1] and Clement Smith's *The Physiology of the Newborn Infant,*[2] both of which appeared in 1946. These classic textbooks made the medical community aware that the neonate and the fetus were deserving of extensive scientific exploration and paved the way for founding the NICUs that began to appear approximately two decades later. Once NICUs came into existence, it was soon appreciated that newborns were an ideal patient group for experimental study. The neonatal period represented a time of life marked by numerous rapid changes that were readily observable; very little was known about either the physiology of newborns or the effect of technology and drugs on their illnesses; and these infants would benefit substantially from the research because so many of them would otherwise not survive. The academic community had, in essence, discovered a gold mine. Consequently, the field of neonatal and perinatal research exploded.

With the rapid expansion of perinatal research during the 1960s and early 1970s, a new phenomenon occurred that was unprecedented in the history of either medicine or medical research. Whereas several years previously it had been generally acknowledged that the neonate was deserving of more research and a greater understanding of his unique physiology, a distinct change developed in the general attitude of health professionals and parents regarding what was an appropriate type of research in general and what was an appropriate amount of research on an individual infant.

These changes in attitude paralleled several important developments including a growing emphasis on human rights and the advent of a better educated and informed public. Furthermore, important changes occurred in the NICU during the late 1970s. Prior to that time, the medical personnel who generally were interested in neonatal or perinatal research were the physicians responsible for the primary care of these infants—mainly neonatologists or obstetricians. Many members of other medical disciplines were skeptical of the value of devoting so much clinical or research time to the newborn infant. It soon became evident, however, that the survival rate of these children was improving, and many academic and private hospitals became anxious to have their own NICUs. Simultaneously, many other subspecialties realized that they were increasingly being consulted about these critically ill infants as well as seeing them in follow-up in various contexts. It was, therefore, only a matter of time before neurologists, hematologists, nephrologists, and others also began asking questions relating to their own disciplines about the neonate. Thus, the newborn, who had previously been the outcast of medicine—with very little attention paid to either patient care or the physiology of transition from fetal to postnatal life—now became the center of attention for all of Pediatrics.

Although this increased attention has unquestionably benefitted individual babies and neonates in general, new problems of major importance have begun to develop. This chapter will focus on selected issues related to these problems and explore various nursing roles in clinical research with the intent of stimulating thought and ultimately enhancing patient care and research interest and involvement.

PRESSURES

In addition to valid scientific reasons to conduct research, many pressures exist that impel the academic researcher to investigate newborn physiology and pathology. The well-known homily of "publish or perish" is a major motivating force in the university community. Academicians who successfully find their way into prestigious journals reap the rewards of advancement in title, increased salary, and enhanced prestige. Also, researchers who use these successes to procure government or private grant money become even more welcome additions to their departments. Thus currently, the newborn is a very desirable but somewhat overstudied commodity. Because so little is known and so much is to be gained, investigators in nearly all fields are anxious to examine the unique attributes of the neonate. The parents of a new baby therefore may be simultaneously approached by several investigators, each eager to utilize the child in a different experiment. Many parents are immediately overwhelmed by such a bombardment of study protocols, either at the time of birth, or on admission of their sick or premature neonate to an NICU.

COUNTER-CURRENT PRESSURES

Recently, both in our hospital—The Children's Hospital of Philadelphia—and in other major neonatal referral centers around the country the questions of what is appropriate research and how much research is appropriate for the individual baby have been asked for the first time. To understand why these questions have surfaced, it is helpful to review some of the factors surrounding birth that make the neonate susceptible to such extensive research.

Typically, the newborn that is part of a research investigation has arrived at this position by one of several ways. Some healthy fullterm infants are studied from a biochemical or physiologic point of view. The main emphasis of these studies is usually the transition from fetal to neonatal life. Illness in the newborn frequently represents an aberration in the physiologic transformation from fetus to neonate. In addition, it may demonstrate the phase during human life when certain physiologic changes can be observed in their purest form.

More commonly, however, the research candidate is either a prematurely born or critically ill neonate admitted to the intensive care nursery of a major hospital or medical center. Thus, in many instances, it is precisely this illness that makes the baby so interesting to so many people.

Because the child is unable to speak for himself and to decide whether or not to participate in a proposed study, the parents of the baby are generally entrusted to make a reasonably intelligent decision regarding his participation. If the parents have a simple clear explanation of what is being evaluated or tested and what the risks and the potential benefits are to the child, making a decision to allow or deny participation appears to be a simple process. In essence, this is the concept of informed consent that has been carefully worked out in painstaking detail to provide the greatest possible protection for the human subject at any age. In practice, however, the process frequently works less smoothly. The reasons why informed consent breaks down in the neonatal period are noteworthy.

ETHICAL DILEMMAS IN INFORMED CONSENT

Prior to the institution of guidelines during the 1970s, it was possible to perform virtually any type of human study, without any regulations controlling the explanation to the experimental subjects of either the purposes of the study or the risks that might result from participation in it. Frequently, inducements such as free medical care or financial rewards would be offered to entice an adequate number of subjects into the protocol. This increased the likelihood that an unscrupulous investigator would perform a somewhat less than ethical study. The neonate was obviously at even greater risk, since he could not speak for himself and it was easy for an investigator to perform a study away from the watchful eye of the child's parents. Thus, with the increase in neonatal research, it became clear that measures were necessary to ensure the safety of the newborn infant.

Fortunately, during this era the National Institutes of Health developed a series of mandatory guidelines for investigators applying for grants. The National Research Act (Pub. L. 93–348, signed into law on July 12, 1974) created the National Commission for the Protection of Human Subjects of Biomedical and Behavioral Research. This act also provided for establishment of review boards at the institutional level—local university, hospital, or other such setting—whose duty it was to safeguard the individual participant by evaluating the type of research being conducted and the ethics of that research. After passage of this act, investigators were obligated to submit both their research protocols and the forms that they were planning to use to obtain informed consent to the Institutional Review Board for evaluation before they began any series of human experiments. Thus, an important measure was added to guarantee that no individual—especially one unable to answer for himself— would be subjected to undue risks.

The subject of informed consent in its entirety is highly complicated—with many legal ramifications—and goes beyond the theme of this chapter.[3] Certain relevant issues, however, are central to the topic of ethical dilemmas in neonatal–perinatal research and merit discussion.

It is clear that parents have a right to know what is being done to their child and why. That concept is one of the basic principles of informed consent for minors. However, from the investigator's point of view, the entire process of obtaining informed consent from parents of a newborn infant is fraught with serious difficulties. First, many types of research that are performed in neonates are so complicated that it is almost beyond the scope of the average parent's level of education to understand the intentions, methods, or risks of the attempted research, no matter how clearly they are explained. The technologic innovations that have been so evident in the NICU are often difficult for even house officers and nurses to comprehend initially. Imagine what the parent confronted with one or several research protocols involving this equipment must attempt to evaluate. Second, because of the very nature of the neonatal period, many phenomena that are crucial to understanding the change from fetal to neonatal life occur so early and are so transient in nature that there is often no time to get informed consent. For example, if one wishes to study the process of initiation of respiration in premature babies, it is often impossible to ask the parents ahead of time for their informed consent and to explain the risks and possible benefits to them. In such cases, the primary built-in safeguard is the Institutional Review Board. Often, if the Board believes that a study has significant merits and is of reasonably low risk to the child, it will approve the study and agree to forego the requirement of obtaining informed consent. However, such instances are relatively unique, and the investigator usually must attempt to secure their informed consent from the parents prior to the baby's birth.

For the parent, the whole research issue is very problematic. Few parents ever expect anything to go wrong during pregnancy, labor, or the delivery of their child. Therefore, when an abnormality does arise, it is frequently a shattering, overwhelming event. Yet this event may be precisely the set of circumstances in which an individual investigator is most interested. Thus, he or she is very anxious to obtain the parents' consent to perform the study that has been painstakingly devised; in contrast, the grief-stricken parents often could not care less about research at this time. These parents who are worried about their critically ill infant may be faced with a number of investigators attempting to explain the ramifications of their studies—the methods, risks, and benefits—all of which may be meaningless to this mother and father. The parents really wish to know only if their child will survive and survive intact. Thus, they often acquiese to their baby's participation in the study in the hope that his survival will somehow be better assured. The converse also may run through their thoughts—that if they refuse to participate, their child may not in some way receive the care that would have been given had they agreed to enroll the baby in the research. Therefore, even though the investigator explains the options clearly and does not attempt to coerce the parents in any way, the parents may strongly believe that enrollment is essential to their baby's well-being. I (A.S.) have had parents urge me to use an unproved, experimental therapy or drug proposed by another investigator, even when I clearly stated to them that I did not believe that the therapy would have any beneficial effects whatsoever, and might, in fact, have some deleterious side-effects. Such responses, which arise from the deep devotion that mothers and fathers often have for their children, virtually from the moment of conception, unfortunately, may invalidate informed consent and lead to inadequate protection for the child. One might appropriately ask at this point if the attempt to study the child under these circumstances is inappropriate and the experiment should be abandoned. Although this course is most likely the prudent one, it is unquestionably difficult for the investigator to react this way, when so many pressures exist for the research to be done.

Other issues of informed consent are equally unclear in this age group. For example, when one approaches a woman at risk for premature delivery to obtain informed consent, can the topics discussed during that conversation—such as the risks to the baby and the problems of prematurity—so stress the mother that the discussion itself actually precipitates the premature birth? Can parents confronted by several different researchers, all asking for informed consent, lose confidence in the ability of the doctors to care for their baby? After all, if the doctors understood how to care for the baby, they wouldn't need to study so many issues, would they? Parents often express such real concerns, and one is forced to wonder whether informed consent protects or interferes with the baby's care.

Finally, from the parents' point of view, research may be a "dirty" word. It is occasionally interpreted to mean that their sick child serves as a guinea pig for an investigator who does not really care for the well-being of their baby but is concerned only with that aspect of care that is part of the experiment. Thus, no matter how clearly it is explained to them, parents may believe that an experiment is undesirable and unnecessary. Some parents consider the word "study" to be less threatening and offensive than "experiment" or "manipulate."[4,5] Terms such as "simple" and "routine" should also be avoided because procedures and techniques that seem simple and routine to the investigator may not appear so to the parent.[5] Thus, the choice of words and manner of presentation may strongly influence parental decision for or against study participation.

In such an atmosphere, then, there is never any true informed consent. The questions being researched are usually too difficult for the mother and father to grasp, and the concepts, no matter how simply described in the informed consent form, are often beyond the reach of even the college-educated parent. Moreover, an oversimplified explanation may change the meaning of informed consent. The time at which informed consent is obtained is one of great stress and duress for the parents, such that their ability to make an intelligent and rational decision and cope with its ramifications is less than ideal. Although they always want the best for the baby, they can never be sure if the proposed study is in their child's best interest. Although many parents recognize the need for research, most of them believe that research is something best done on someone else or someone else's baby. Thus, the parents of the neonate often have major unresolvable dilemmas when confronted with the request to allow their infant or multiple-birth infants to participate in one or several studies.

NURSING AND NEONATAL RESEARCH— CHANGING ATTITUDES

The substantial increase in perinatal research in the past several years has posed numerous ethical and attitudinal problems for the obstetrical and the neonatal nurse. Neonatology, has been particularly exemplified by a dramatic shift in care techniques, so that the time-honored philosophy of leaving the critically ill neonate alone as much as possible has been replaced by a need to coordinate the sophisticated equipment used to monitor his progress. Such coordination efforts necessitate that the babies are handled more frequently. However, introduction of the transcutaneous oxygen ($TcPO_2$) electrode has demonstrated that the older philosophy may not necessarily have been bad. This device has demonstrated that even minor manipulations of the sick neonate result in major drops in $TcPO_2$ levels. Incorporating this knowledge into nursing practice to limit the number of times and the manner in which the infant is handled may create an almost immediate conflict between the NICU nurse and the investigator. Other concerns may also create dilemmas. A frequently occurring example is the realization that the study may cause some—it is hoped, transient—effects on the baby that may not be beneficial and may in fact be somewhat harmful. This ethical concern, however, conflicts with a professional orientation that acknowledges the need for research to improve the overall care that many babies receive. Situations like these create definite dilemmas for the nurse in regard to her role in research in the NICU.

Besides ethical concerns and the question of how much the sick neonate should be disturbed for the purpose of study, neonatal research creates many other burdens. The nurse often finds that various projects interfere with the ability to perform nursing functions. Physical obstacles such as special test equipment and the presence of extra research personnel impede access to the infant, the chart, and flowsheets. Research imposes additional tasks such as collecting specimens; administering medications; monitoring, documenting and communicating effects of study procedures; transcribing extra orders; learning new protocols; relating to more people; and planning the work day around the demands of the protocol. Since the timing of care and procedures in the NICU is in a very delicate balance, the nurse must frequently reorganize and sacrifice so that the needs of both patient and investigator can be met. Occasionally, the demands of the study schedule may supercede the priorities of patient care—ranging from basic care to treating sudden deterioration to the need to be with a parent. Thus an intellectual conflict may occur. Another situation may be stressful as well as an imposition. The nurse is often the only person in attendance during certain phases of the study. Therefore, parents frequently ask the nurse to describe and clarify the meaning of the project. They also ask the nurse to share his/her views and feelings with them about the particular study(ies) and about research in general.

Added to the well-documented stresses of the NICU, these burdens may be more than the individual nurse can handle. The mixed feelings about the research that is being conducted, the critical timing for data collection, the increased amount, complexity, and obstacles of the workload and the need for its frequent reorganization, the concern for the welfare of the parents at such a stressful time and the pointed questions that they ask—especially if the nurse does not feel confident and comfortable discussing the studies—may lead to an inability to cope in an already difficult environment. Therefore, it is of utmost importance that the investigator weave the neonatal nurse into the study design in such a way as to create a belief that the added responsibility and stresses posed by the investigation are indeed worthwhile and that the study is a reasonable risk for the infant and parent.

Several measures can be undertaken to enhance the knowledge, attitudes, and cooperation of the interdisciplinary staff providing care in the nursery. Institutional research philosophies (both medical and nursing) and the responsibilities of medical, nursing, and other personnel should be introduced and clarified in employment interviews and orientation sessions. However, two corollaries follow. If nursing employment is accepted without clearly defined expectations of research activities and responsibilities, the nurse should have the option of not participating in research.[6] Furthermore, personnel cannot be expected to engage in a study that violates their own ethical or moral principles.[6] Thus, the concept of informed consent also applies to medical personnel. It is important, though, that the neonatal nurse who takes a position in a university-based tertiary-level nursery understands that such units have more than the simple obligation to provide the best care for the sick newborn. These NICUs are also obligated to perform research of the highest caliber to benefit all sick neonates.

Other measures such as ongoing inservices and conferences on current research projects, preferably given by the principal investigator, are especially beneficial. In addition to explaining the primary objective of the study, sessions should include the potential effects that the project may have on nursing and medical care, the responsibilities of the research team and nursery staff, and the communication network. At such sessions, the nursery staff should be encouraged to discuss their misgivings about the research and to question any aspect of the study that they do not understand or that they believe is potentially detrimental to the outcome of the infant and/or the family. These meetings should also be used as sensitivity sessions to allow venting of feelings and active staff participation in resolving concerns such as the parent's welfare at a time of high stress and frustrations such as burdensome workloads and loss of control of patient management that are sometimes perceived by nurses and residents. These sessions serve to acknowledge difficult situations, allow staff to verbalize concerns and validate perceptions in a supportive environment even though resolutions may not be possible, discuss alternatives and solicit problem-solving ideas, and emphasize that research is relatively short-term compared with the benefits of the expected outcome. The nursery staff may also provide the investigator with improved methods of conducting the research. Often, these sessions may readily defuse issues or misconceptions that lead to conflict between nurse, parents, and investigator. As a corollary, the staff should be provided with the results of the study once all the data have been collected and analyzed and informed of infant status at follow-up visits. This simple courtesy earns respect for the researcher, increases the staff's knowledge, and fosters further collaborative efforts.

Additional measures like periodic bedside discussions about the study(ies) in which the infant is enrolled are also helpful. A standardized research manual of studies currently in progress in the NICU that includes protocols, descriptions, goals, dates of projects, study personnel, responsibilities, and particular information such as commonly asked questions and answers about the project or topic being investigated provides a resource for frequently changing staff, students, and nursery visitors. A research nurse or associate actively involved in the NICU can enhance knowledge regarding the research process, particular studies, communication, and collaboration—which acts to preserve the integrity of protocols. These approaches will readily bring the nursing staff into the research being conducted, allay anxiety related to research, and enable the nurse to deal better with parent questions regarding methods, effects, and results of the studies in progress (see Chapter 10, Section on Communication).

NURSING ROLES IN CLINICAL RESEARCH

Research activity and the utilization of knowledge are responsibilities of each practitioner. (Murphy K; personal communication). Furthermore, each nurse has the responsibility to educate. Since parents with infants who require intensive care situations often develop closer bonds to their nurses than to their physicians, the neonatal nurse can help to educate parents and allay their misgivings by demonstrating a sensitive and positive attitude and by explaining various aspects of research. Information may include an emphasis on the newness of neonatology, the means by which therapy is being evaluated on a daily basis, the numerous ways that studies benefit infants now and in the future, and a discussion of specific questions asked by the parents about the study(ies) in which their infant is enrolled.

Many institutions utilize the concept of primary nursing that holds the primary nurse responsible and accountable for the total nursing care of her patients throughout hospitalization. Generally, components of the primary nurse's role include responsibility for direct patient care, collaboration, consultation, patient advocacy, and health teaching. Institutional requirements for specific duties vary. Most of the following thoughts relate to this author's (K.S.M.) views on current and potential nursing roles in clinical research. Many of these qualities and activities are evident today.

The primary nurse (PN) is the key person in the clinical setting. She should promote a positive attitude about research and understand the importance of projects and their potential benefit to the patient and nursing and medical management. She is the liaison to associate nurses, medical and research teams, and parents, and she promotes collaborative relationships. The primary nurse knows which infants are enrolled in specific studies and appreciates the value of the projects. She also utilizes resources such as manuals, protocols, flow sheets, and study personnel. The PN is sensitive to nursing conflicts, frustrations, and ethical dilemmas about clinical research, and provides anticipatory guidance for participation in research endeavors. The PN plays an essential role in fostering the integrity and successful outcome of clinical studies.

The research associate (RA), or research nurse, is a valuable contributor to the clinical environment. The stereotypical role in this instance is one of data collector. This role, however, can be substantially expanded to enhance the quality of the research effort. This expanded position is preferably filled by a nurse with graduate training (M.S.N. degree) who has a solid understanding of the research process and is able to translate research findings into clinical practice. The RA may be responsible for a major long-term project or for several smaller projects. This role may require that the RA coordinate, implement, and participate in the project. Additionally, it may involve assisting in analyzing, presenting and publishing the findings, and possibly participating in developing future projects and writing grants.

The nurse-RA gains the confidence and cooperation of the staff through demonstrated credibility in practice, teaching, and interpersonal relationships. She informs nurses, physicians, medical students, and other personnel about assigned projects through both impromptu and planned sessions at the bedside, at conferences, and during daily rounds. She documents clinical findings, provides handouts and literature related to the project to rotating staff, and may be responsible for developing and maintaining the unit's manual of current research projects. The RA promotes public relations and develops a trusting relationship with families of infants enrolled in studies in which she is involved. This role may include clarifying aspects of informed consent and keeping parents informed of their infant's progress throughout a clinical trial.

The RA fosters a sense of inquiry and stimulates assessment and evaluation of findings. Through collaboration and cooperation she helps to minimize excessive manipulation and stresses to the infant. She should also provide feedback on the outcome of particular aspects of the study and of infant follow-up to the nursery staff.

Another expanded role is emerging, that of the neonatal critical care nurse practitioner (NCCNP). Although role expectations may vary from one institution to another, essentially the NCCNP provides primary care in a variety of settings under the direction of—and frequently in the absence of—physicians. The role includes assessing, diagnosing, and performing routine and emergency procedures among many other diverse and important responsibilities. Fulfilling this role will greatly contribute to successful nursing and medical management of the high-risk infant. Although, it is beyond the scope of this chapter to discuss highly charged issues involving the NCCNP such as legal considerations related to Nurse Practice Acts, licensure, and the severe shortage of critical care nurses, the likelihood exists that the NCCNP will be a physician extender. With respect to research and in view of the increasing shortage of medical fellows and housestaff, the NCCNP may become involved in research projects heretofore implemented by physicians. The NCCNP may demonstrate many of the qualities of the RA. It is important to understand that none of the previously described roles are meant to be mutually exclusive. Rather, the roles and capabilities of the individuals in these positions overlap in many aspects.

All of these nursing roles have thus far been described in relation to medical research, because nursing research is not yet widespread. Nursing roles in the context of nursing research differ from the descriptions above in their emphasis on (1) the practitioner's responsibility to identify areas for nursing research, to participate whenever possible, and to utilize the results to improve nursing practice; (2) the responsibility of practitioners with advanced degrees to formulate questions for nursing research and to develop, implement, disseminate, and publish the results; and (3) the distinction that research is not *nursing* research because it is done by a nurse. Nurses who collect data for investigators from other disciplines are not "nurse researchers"; they are data collectors.[7] This last statement is not intended to minimize involvement of nurses in medical research but rather to denote the difference. The previously described role of the RA is important to both medical and nursing practice.

Although there is ongoing debate concerning who is capable of doing research and traditionalists say that only nurses with the doctorate degree qualify, nursing research is currently being conducted by nurses with a commitment to practice, even by staff nurses without formal research training.[7] Collaborative efforts and support make this possible. Moreover, "research does not have to be complicated to be good."[7]

THE FUTURE OF PERINATAL CRITICAL CARE
NURSING AND RESEARCH

During the 1980s, nursing involvement in research and utilization of knowledge will be impressive. Critical care nurses will continue to play a major and changing role in perinatal research by participating in medical, nursing and interdisciplinary projects and by developing and implementing nursing research to validate nursing theory and actions, generate new knowledge, and improve infant and family outcome. Positive institutional and individual philosophies and attitudes coupled with advanced educational preparation will help to promote research and to assure its integrity, successful implementation, and dissemination. Educational preparation will be a key factor. Many new doctoral and some PhD programs will be developed to prepare nurses for research and graduate faculty teaching positions. Of great importance will be the consideration of equivalent programs for advanced practitioners, educators, administrators, and evaluators.[8] Nurses with an MSN degree will contribute greatly to an increased amount of clinical research and its translation to clinical practice. A strong ripple effect will result from an emphasis on research that is already incorporated at the baccalaureate level and from that disseminated in unit conferences, inservice sessions, continuing education programs, and Research Days. The last four modes to promote research are gaining momentum. Other events will occur. These will include developing support systems such as institutional Departments of Nursing Research, hiring nurse researchers to promote and enhance research of nurses, providing joint appointments to link academia and service, and designing feedback loops between *all* levels of nursing.[9]

Critical care nurses are increasingly becoming involved in research at local, regional, and national levels. In 1981 hundreds of nurse experts participated in the first nationwide Delphi Study to Identify Priorities in Critical Care Nursing Research, sponsored by the American Association of Critical-Care Nurses (AACN). An outcome of this study, which concerns 13 subspecialty areas, will be to encourage and promote research according to the stipulated priorities. Critical care nurses in all subspecialities will be encouraged to seek funding. To support further research efforts and provide resources, AACN is currently developing a Nurse Researcher Directory in which nurses are listed according to their areas of research activity and interest. These collective efforts should promote multi-center collaborative nursing research endeavors (Christine Breu, President-Elect, The American Association of Critical-Care Nurses, personal communication). Fostering perinatal education is a major commitment of the Nurses Association of the American College of Obstetricians and Gynecologists (NAACOG). Recent research activities have resulted in published Guidelines for Childbirth Education. Current efforts are being directed toward the publication of a document describing the role and education guidelines for the NICU nurse. Future commitments will probably be directed toward developing and supporting perinatal research efforts (Mary Bolster Wagner, Director, Dept. of Education, NAACOG, personal communication). Both the American Nurses Association (ANA) and Sigma Theta Tau, the National Honor Society of Nursing, are committed to nursing research, and state nursing associations are becoming more committed. A more indepth discussion of organizational involvement in nursing research is beyond the scope of this chapter.

Within the next few decades, significantly more nurses will hold doctorate degrees and will conduct research, and even more nurses will be impressively involved in research. Research support efforts will continue to focus on individual nurse researchers but will shift towards greater support for collaborative relationships, research partnerships, cluster studies, or research consortia.[10] An anticipated outcome will be major grant awards to nurses. Nurses will be known for their research abilities, contributions, and clout, and institutions will be known for their nurses' expertise. Along with these advances, nurses will undoubtedly contribute, be subject to, and help to resolve the above-mentioned trends, pressures, and conflicts associated with perinatal care and growth.

SUMMARY

This chapter has attempted to outline some of the current problems that are unique to perinatal research. Many ethical and technical difficulties currently exist that provide excellent opportunities for nursing involvement, organization, and education. It is clear that such opportunities require nursing interaction at many different levels to help guide parents and infants through the research process. Several role models have been described, but these are only a starting point. It is hoped that with continued growth in neonatal and perinatal research, the role of the nurse will also expand to fill new and unforeseen situations. Such an evolution will certainly lead to new, highly satisfying careers in this essential field of nursing.

REFERENCES

1. Barcroft Sir Joseph: Researches in Pre-Natal Life. Oxford, England, Blackwell Scientific, 1946
2. Smith CA: The Physiology of the Newborn Infant. Springfield, IL, Charles C Thomas, 1946
3. Cassileth BR, Zupkis RV, Sutton-Smith K, March V: Informed consent—why are its goals imperfectly realized? N Engl J Med 302:896, 1980
4. Owens J: An overview of nursing research. Lecture presented at conference sponsored by the Southeastern Pennsylvania Chapter of the American Association of Critical-Care Nurses, Philadelphia, May 14, 1980
5. Hayter J: Issues related to human subjects. In: Issues in Nursing Research. eds. Downs FS and Fleming JW. New York, Appleton-Century-Crofts, 1979, pp 107–147
6. American Nurses Association: Human Rights Guidelines for Nurses in Clinical and Other Research. Kansas City, MO, American Nurses Association, 1975
7. Hodgman EC: Closing the gap between research and practice: changing the answers to the "who," the "where," and the "how" of nursing research. Int J Nurs Stud 16:105, 1979
8. Cleland V: Educational issues related to research in nursing. In: Issues in Nursing Research. eds. Downs FS and Fleming JW. New York, Appleton-Century-Crofts, 1979, pp 25–38
9. Fleming JW: The future of nursing research. In: Issues in Nursing Research. eds. Downs FS and Fleming JW. New York, Appleton-Century-Crofts, 1979, pp 149–178
10. Stevenson JS: Support for an emerging social institution. In: Issues in Nursing Research. eds. Downs FS and Fleming JW. New York, Appleton-Century-Crofts, 1979, pp 39–66

SUGGESTED READING

American Association of Critical-Care Nurses: Compilation of Research Abstracts for Critical Care Nurses, 1st edn, ed. Irvine CA. American Association of Critical-Care Nurses, 1976

American Association of Critical-Care Nurses: Compilation of Research Abstracts for Critical Care Nurses, 2nd edn, ed. Irvine CA. American Association of Critical-Care Nurses, 1979

Barnard K: Knowledge for practice: directions for the future. Nurs Res 29:208, 1980

Breu C, Dracup K: Implementing nursing research in a critical care setting. J Nurs Adm 6:14, 1976

Ciske KL: Primary nursing: an organization that promotes professional practice. J Nurs Adm 4:29, 1975

Davis M: Promoting research in the clinical setting. J Nurs Adm 11:22, 1981

Downs FS: Relationship of findings of clinical research and development of criteria: a researcher's perspective. Nurs Res 19:94, 1980

Fawcett J: A declaration of nursing independence: the relation of theory and research to nursing practice. J Nurs Adm 10:36, 1980

Fleming JW, Hayter J: Reading research reports critically. Nurs Outlook 22:172, 1974

Fuhs MF, Moore K: Research program development in a tertiary care setting. Nurs Res 30:24, 1981

Hodgman EC: Student research in service agencies. Nurs Outlook 26:558, 1978

Hodgman EC: Research policy for nursing services: part I. J Nurs Adm 11:30, 1981

Hodgman EC: Research policy for nursing services: Part II. J Nurs Adm 11:33, 1981

Jacox A, Prescott P: Determining a study's relevance for clinical practice. AJN 78:1882, 1978

Jacox A: Strategies to promote nursing research. Nurs Res 29:213, 1980

Kelly K, McClelland E: Signed consent: protection or constraint? Nurs Outlook 27:40, 1979

Ketefian S: Problems in the dissemination and utilization of knowledge: how can the gap be bridged? In: Translation of Theory into Nursing Practice and Education. with a Bibliography on Change. ed. Ketefian S. New York, New York University, Division of Nursing, 1975

King D, Barnard K, Hoehn R: Disseminating the results of nursing research. Nurs Outlook 29:164, 1981

Kreuger J: Nursing administrators' roles in research: the WICHE program. Nurs Adm Q 2:27, 1978

Larson E: The inquisitive nurse: bringing research to the bedside. Nurs Adm Q 2:9, 1978

Mancini M: Consent to treatment: what does it entail? AJN 79:1139, 1979

McLaughlin, FE: The publication of nursing research. J Nurs Adm 11:37, 1981

Misner SJ: Nursing research: key to a locked-in profession. Supervisor Nurse 8:37, 1977

Paletta JL: Nursing research: an integral part of professional nursing. Image 12:3–6, 1980

Protecting research subjects. AJN 79:1139, 1979

Robb SS: Nurse involvement in institutional review boards: The service setting perspective. Nurs Res 30:27, 1981

Stetler CB, Marram G: Evaluating research findings for applicability in practice. Nurs Outlook 24:559, 1976

Ward MJ, Fetler ME: Research report evaluation checklist. Nurs Res 28:120, 1979

6 The Child with Chronic Respiratory Failure: A Special Challenge

Barbara D. Schraeder
Mary E. Donar

Children who survive acute respiratory failure but remain dependent on ventilatory assistance for their survival present new and complex challenges to the intensive care nurse. Although actual statistics on the number of such children are sparse and poorly documented, personal communications from nurses nationwide suggest that there is scarcely an infant or pediatric intensive care unit that has not had the experience of caring for a child with this perplexing problem. The child's precarious physical state, the long-term nature of his illness with its uncertain outcome, the frustration and anxiety experienced by the child's family, and the extraordinary financial and professional investment challenge nurses to use all dimensions of their nursing science and art. This chapter focuses on two major areas—the care of the child with chronic respiratory failure specifically resulting from chronic lung disease and the issues related to this care. The population of children involved and the social and organizational aspects of the phenomenon are discussed. The chapter also identifies specific nursing diagnosis, intervention, and evaluation strategies and describes the nurse as caregiver, coordinator, and "significant other."

CHRONIC RESPIRATORY FAILURE OF INFANCY

Chronic respiratory failure of infancy (CRFI) is a newly described pediatric disease state. Children with this syndrome are dependent on mechanical ventilators and tracheostomies and are resistant to traditional methods of weaning from respiratory support.

The syndrome has two primary causes. The first is a neuromuscular dysfunction that interferes with the child's ability to move air effectively in and out of the lungs. This category includes both hereditary neuromuscular disorders—e.g., Werdnig-Hoffman's disease, Duchenne dystrophy, the myotubular myopathies—and acquired neuromuscular dysfunction such as infantile botulism and cervical cord transection. The muscle weakness or dysfunction leads to a state of hypoventilation, hypercapnea, and atelectasis. Chronic infection and pneumonia become superimposed on what was initially a mechanical problem.

The second primary cause of CRFI is chronic lung alteration that severely interferes with pulmonary dynamics. Such chronic lung changes are grouped under the name of bronchopulmonary dysplasia (BPD). This type of dysplasia typically affects the smallest, most fragile premature infants who have been treated for respiratory disorders with endotracheal intubation, prolonged positive pressure ventilation, and high concentrations of inspired oxygen.[1-3] BPD is also found in fullterm infants who have had severe meconium aspiration syndrome, tracheo-esophageal fistulas, congenital heart disease, and congenital anomalies of the chest wall.[4]

Respiratory failure is defined as chronic if the infant needs ventilatory support for more than 3 months despite repeated attempts to wean that use traditional methods.[5-7] Chronic respiratory failure has three possible outcomes: (1) the child dies because increasing levels of support fail to provide adequate ventilation; (2) the condition is stabilized but is refractory to any weaning programs, and the child is able to live indefinitely with respiratory assistance; and (3) the child is successfully weaned after a program of support that is sensitive to his total well-being, and he is able to live free of respiratory assistance. To understand the evolution of CRFI, it is important to identify the anatomic and physiologic peculiarities of the infant's respiratory system and to review the underlying pathophysiology of bronchopulmonary dysplasia.

Anatomy and Physiology of the Infant's Respiratory System

During fetal development the lung is functionally inactive, but it undergoes extensive anatomic and histologic differentiation after birth. Normally, these structural and physiologic changes continue through infancy and childhood and into adolescence. Alveolarization occurs throughout childhood, and the full adult complement of alveoli is almost achieved by 8 years of age. The alveoli begin to increase in size at approximately age 5 but are not fully mature until adolescence. After adolescence they have the concentration, density, and elastic fiber characteristic of adult alveoli.[8]

The infant's lung compliance is half that of the adult, but airway resistance is 15–17 times greater. Because the infant's overall metabolic rate is double that of the adult, he must invest a greater proportion of calories per kilogram to move air in and out of his lungs. Consequently, anything that increases airway resistance places tremendous demands on a system with minimal reserve function.[9]

Incidence and Pathophysiology of Chronic Respiratory Failure of Infancy

Bronchopulmonary dysplasia is a generalized lung disease that involves all structures of the lung. In some children, the reserve is stressed to such an extent that chronic respiratory failure ensues. The syndrome was first described by Northway et al. in 1967.[10]

The incidence of chronic lung disease secondary to BPD seems to vary from center to center probably because of both the lack of agreement on diagnostic criteria and the differing natures of infant intensive care units (IICUs). It has been suggested that the disease is more prevalent in major referral centers that receive infants who are born at local or community hospitals and then subjected to the hazards of being transported to the IICU. Reports of occurrence range from 7–68% in survivors of positive pressure ventilation.[11,12] The percentage of infants that remain ventilator-dependent for prolonged periods of time is not well-documented. A report of pediatric surgical patients who received ventilatory support during a 3-year period, 1975–1978, indicates that 3.5% (13 children) required prolonged support (100 or more days). The range was 101–1,240 days, with a mean of 359 days and a median of 278 days. Survival was 42%.[5] A second report from the same institution described 32 children who had CRFI during the years 1974–1979. Survival in this group was 72%.[6]

Children with BPD have diffuse, obliterative airway disease, interstitial fibrosis and persistent collapse of portions of the lung, partial lung atrophy, diminished alveolarization, and evidence of pulmonary hypertension.[3] The following scenario may lead to CRFI.[13] A susceptible infant develops hypoxemia and acidosis and may also be hypothermic, hypovolemic, and hypoglycemic. Oxygen therapy is initiated or is increased for continued venous admixture, and at the same time the infant is warmed, and buffers, plasma expanders, transfusions, and glucose infusions are administered. However, when the cells have been damaged by hypoxia, those in the bronchioles and alveolar ducts slough, and the denuded areas fill with a high-protein fluid. Successful therapy replaces pulmonary vasoconstriction with pulmonary vasodilation, including dilation of the capillaries. The alveolar spaces fill with fluid because the lymphatic system is inadequate to remove the interstitial fluid. At this time ventilatory assistance is usually initiated or increased, and the resultant increased airway pressure on the fluid-filled terminal conducting airways frequently forces air into the interstitium. This air migrates into the peribronchial and perivascular lymphatics and causes a pneumothorax or pneumomediastinum. Chest tubes are put in place, higher airway pressures are needed for adequate ventilation, and the percentage of inspired oxygen is increased.

The lymphatic vessels (now filled with air) cannot clear the fluid and pulmonary edema results. The consequential hypoxemia leads to a left-to-right shunt through the ductus arteriosus. Airway pressure and oxygen are increased to deal with the new complication. The high inspired oxygen concentration destroys the pulmonary cells and creates a diffusion barrier because of the large areas of damaged lung tissue. Retention of CO_2 occurs because of increasing dead-space ventilation. Pressure damages the conducting airways and the supporting tissues. Collagen production becomes excessive in an attempt to repair the lung that has become stiff and overdistended. A low-grade infection (usually) from pseudomonas aeruginosa or aerobacter klebsiella is acquired. The infant is now ventilator dependent and is hypercarbic and hypoxemic.[13]

Diagnosis is based on radiographic and clinical criteria. The radiographic evidence has been differentiated into four stages.[10]

Stage I.   The period of acute respiratory distress syndrome. X-ray films of the lungs reveal the presence of widespread alveolar atelectasis, air bronchograms, hyaline membranes, and hyperemia. Lymphatic dilation is present.

Stage II.   The period of regeneration, seen on days 4–10. Both lung fields are completely opacified and the cardiac border is obscured.

Stage III.   The period of transition to chronic disease, seen on days 10–20. On X-ray, the lungs have areas of irregular density and a spongy appearance, and bullae are present.

Stage IV.   The period of chronic disease, seen after one month. On X-ray the lung has a spongy appearance and cardiomegaly is present. Clinically the child appears cyanotic and has fine diffuse râles on auscultation.

Diagnosis and Medical Approaches to Care

The clinical diagnosis of BPD is based on the following criteria.

1.   Intermittent positive pressure ventilation is required during the first week of life, for a minimum of 3 days

2.   Clinical signs of chronic respiratory disease characterized by tachypnea, intercostal and subcostal retractions, and râles on auscultation are present and persist for longer than 28 days

3.   Supplemental O_2 to maintain a PaO_2 greater than 50 torr is needed for more than 28 days

4.   The chest X-ray shows persistant strands of densities in both lungs, alternating with areas of normal and increased lucency; these larger areas resemble bullae[13,14]

The clinical signs and symptoms associated with CRFI secondary to late-stage BPD are hyperinflation of the lungs, tachypnea, wheezing, cyanotic episodes, excessive work of breathing accompanied by hypercapnea, pulmonary arterial hypertension with increased pulmonary vascular resistance, inappropriate water retention (especially in the lungs), and recurrent pulmonary infection.[15] The infants are dependent on mechanical ventilation with tracheostomy for survival.[8] They show signs of growth retardation and developmental delay,[14-16] and most remain below the 3rd percentile in height and weight. They tend to have a large head size relative to trunk size—a possible consequence of hypoxia or of obstructed venous return during positive-pressure ventilation.[16]

Pulmonary function in children with chronic respiratory failure is characterized by decreased dynamic compliance, increased airway resistance, increased physiologic dead space, and an increase in the pulmonary venous admixture.[15] A study of the breathing patterns in seven infants (ages 3–16 months) who were dependent on mechanical ventilation because of BPD revealed the presence of elevated lower airway resistance, a low dynamic lung compliance, and a rapid respiratory rate when compared with normal values. The end-tidal CO_2 tension (PCO_2) was elevated in spite of abnormally high minute ventilation. The study suggested that weaning from ventilatory support was concommitant with the ability to sustain a high minute volume in spite of persistently elevated airway resistance and low dynamic lung compliance.[16,17]

The ability to sustain high minute volumes in spite of persistently elevated airway resistance and low dynamic compliance seems to be related to the child's growth and development with the accompanying increase in strength and vigor.[16] Consequently, recovery depends on adequate nutrition, the control or the minimizing of occurrences of infection, and the provision of adequate respiratory support. The last factor is particularly important, because there is evidence that chronic hypoxemia, in addition to weakening the child and compromising his ability to resist infection, may lead to constriction of the pulmonary vascular bed and fixed pulmonary hypertension.[18] With adequate supportive care, gas exchange improves and growth and development occur, leading to increased strength in the diaphragmatic and accessory respiratory muscles. With the increasing size, strength, and vigor, dynamic lung compliance increases and the previously elevated lower airway resistance is decreased, allowing the infant to compensate for his high dead-space ventilation.[16]

Therefore, the long-term medical goal of weaning from respiratory support is accomplished by the following activities:

1. Controlling and minimizing respiratory infections and insults that compromise the healing and growing potential of the maturing lung
2. Maximizing gas diffusion across the alveolar membrane to keep the child in an optimal respiratory state with the smallest amount of potentially damaging respiratory support
3. Ensuring that nutrition is adequate to support the growth of the tra-

cheal-bronchial tree and to improve the strength of the accessory muscles of breathing

4. Providing optimal cardiopulmonary assistance with minimal damage to the tracheal-bronchial structure

Medical interventions can be divided into three parameters: pharmacologic therapy; surveillance and treatment of infection, and ventilatory assistance with a carefully directed program of weaning.

Pharmacologic interventions are directed at improving gas exchange and cardiac functioning. Children who require long-term mechanical ventilation retain fluid, particularly in the interstitial spaces of the lung. Fluid retention is characteristic of chronic lung disease of infancy, but evidence suggests that it is also a common side effect of mechanical ventilation.[19] Restricting water and initiating diuretic therapy improve the infant's ability to ventilate and to utilize oxygen. Pulmonary fluid retention causes respiratory compromise by increasing the work of breathing and by changing lung compliance, thus increasing both ventilation and oxygen requirements. Consequently, the child often requires a regimen of diuretic therapy supplemented with electrolytes. Three diuretics—chlorothiazide, spironolactone, and furosemide—are commonly used alone or in combination to produce diuresis. Electrolyte replacement must be carefully monitored to prevent electrolyte imbalance and to enhance the optimal effect of the diuretics. The long-term effects of diuretic therapy in young infants are unknown, but medical practice suggests that the benefits outweigh the risks.

Another group of drugs that enhance pulmonary function in chronic lung disease of infancy are the aminophylline derivatives.[20,21] Infants treated with mechanical ventilation and high concentrations of oxygen have higher than normal amounts of bronchiolar smooth muscle. The muscle is swollen and hypertrophied and contributes to the high airway resistance. In infants 3 months of age and younger theophylline decreases airway resistance, increases dynamic compliance, and improves the distribution of ventilation by relaxing the smooth muscles of the airways.[22] Maintenance doses are useful in optimizing pulmonary function and seem to have a mild diuretic effect.[21]

Digitalis derivatives may also be used when right ventricular hypertrophy is present to enhance cardiac output and improve cardiac functioning.[20]

Surveillance for and prompt treatment of infection are important medical interventions. The child's tracheostomy bypasses the respiratory tract's normal mechanisms for defense against infection. This is aggravated by the inability to cough spontaneously and the repeated introduction of foreign bodies into the tracheal–bronchial tree for suctioning of secretions. Additionally, the child's chronically debilitated state makes him a susceptible host to a variety of viral and bacterial infections. Acute viral infections may become protracted and be complicated by secondary bacterial infections.[23] It is imperative to identify the pathogen quickly and institute appropriate treatment.

The third area of medical treatment is respiratory care and weaning from ventilatory support. Successful weaning can take place in the hospital or in the home after the child is discharged. Criteria for the latter alternative include the following:

1. The availability of concerned and well-motivated caregivers
2. Respiratory stability on current levels of support as defined by (a) a positive trend on growth curves, (b) stamina for periods of play, (c) relative freedom from successive bouts of respiratory infection and fever, and (d) maintenance of a partial arterial pressure of oxygen (PaO_2) of 60–90 torr and a partial arterial pressure of carbon dioxide ($PaCO_2$) of 45–50 torr
3. The presence of an adequate physical environment at home
4. The availability of financial support from third party payers
5. The provision of service, supplies, and equipment on an on-going basis

Weaning at home appears to be a successful and financially sound alternative to hospital care for some children.[5,7] Whether at home or in the hospital, weaning is a slow, meticulous process that encompasses the totality of the child's physiologic, social, and emotional well-being. It involves changing only one or two parameters at a time, frequently at weekly or bi-weekly intervals. It may mean that the child remains at minimally toxic settings until physical growth and development permit him to achieve enough strength to compensate for the damaged lung tissue. Appropriate weaning requires that the medical practitioner modify the usual rapid approach to weaning and exercise patience and sensitivity to the child's response.

NURSING CARE OF THE CHILD WITH CRFI

Professional nursing care that is based on a holistic approach to the child and his family is a major factor in securing a positive outcome for the child with CRFI. All children with this difficult problem have, or are at risk for, four major nursing diagnoses: (1) altered respiratory state; (2) altered nutritional state, (3) altered sensori-motor development, and (4) altered family relationships.

Altered Respiratory State

Consistent, on-going nursing observation and intervention are essential in respiratory management for the child with CRFI. The goal of respiratory care is to provide an environment in which the immature respiratory system can develop optimally. Such development and the child's eventual recovery depend on adequate respiratory support, control of infection, and adequate nutrition. Experience has shown that these goals are interrelated, because weaning from respiratory support cannot occur without a steady rate of growth and the control of infection.[24]

Nursing care that is directed toward ensuring an optimal environment for recovery includes (1) on-going assessment of respiratory functioning by clinical evaluations and non-invasive and invasive monitoring techniques; (2) supportive respiratory therapy; (3) assessment of the patient's potential for being weaned; (4) evaluation of the weaning program; and (5) surveillance for and prevention of infection.

Clinical Assessment of Respiratory Function. Careful observation is the foundation of clinical assessment of the child with CRFI. The vital signs, especially the respiratory rate, are accurate indicators of overall respiratory state and tolerance of support. Other important parameters are skin color (especially in response to stressful situations), respiratory effort and chest wall movement; quality and equality of breath sounds as heard on auscultation; and quantity, quality, and color of tracheal secretions. A flow sheet documenting chest assessment and the character of secretions enhances the value of clinical observations by providing the earliest suggestion of a developing infection.

Non-Invasive Techniques for Assessing Respiratory Function. Non-invasive monitoring procedures include transcutaneous oxygen monitoring, end-tidal capnography, and impedence pneumography. Non-invasive techniques are preferred in long-term care for the well-being of the child, since frequent measurements are necessary. Although the accuracy of the information obtained via noninvasive monitoring is not absolute, consistent use provides reliable value ranges and trends.

The transcutaneous PO_2 ($TcPO_2$) monitor is used to evaluate oxygen status. Initially, the accuracy of the $TcPO_2$ reading should be confirmed with an arterial blood-gas sample. Once this value has been established, $TcPO_2$ monitoring can be used to spot-check oxygenation and provide information on PO_2 changes in response to stress (Kettrick RG: unpublished abstract). The oxygen concentration that is delivered can then be adjusted to maintain an acceptable $TcPO_2$. It has been noted that the response time of the $TcPO_2$ monitor is slightly faster with decreasing than with increasing PO_2.[25] Although the numbers are not always accurate, the $TcPO_2$ readings may compare closely with the PO_2, with variable increases in $TcPO_2$ noted in response to increased skin temperature and decreases noted with oxygen consumption by the tissues.[26]

End-tidal capnography to evaluate CO_2 has recently become available for routine clinical care. When accuracy is confirmed with an arterial blood gas, capnography is used to monitor the adequacy of alveolar ventilation. The correlation between end-tidal CO_2 ($ETCO_2$) and PCO_2 in children has been shown to be excellent.[27]

With proper application and observation, the hazards of $TcPO_2$ monitoring are minimal. The nurse can prevent skin site burns from the $TCPO_2$ electrode by routinely changing the electrodes.

An impedence pneumograph, with its built-in alarm, provides continuous monitoring of respiratory rate. It may also be used to indicate tachypnea. However, its principal value for the often active child with an artificial airway is that it increases safety, because it indicates apnea resulting from obstruction or decannulation.

Invasive Techniques for Assessing Respiratory Function. Invasive monitoring via arterial blood gas (ABG) levels is a highly traumatic procedure for the alert and active child. Attempts should be made to avoid this procedure. ABG levels should be ascertained (1) for initial confirmation of non-invasive measurements, (2) if necessary during an acute process, and (3) when the dependability of the $TcPO_2$ and $ETCO_2$ measurements is doubtful. Every effort should be made to comfort the child during and after the procedure. Infants can often be distracted if offered a pacifier. Soothing words and the presence of the nurse often provide comfort to the older child. Administering a local anesthetic to the arterial puncture site can both lessen the child's discomfort and increase the accuracy of the value. Although the child may be uncomfortable during injection of the anesthetic into the skin, he will often be calm while the blood is obtained.

Supportive Respiratory Therapy.   The nurse has an integral part in maintaining the quality of supportive respiratory therapy. Humidification of the airway must be ensured by carefully checking respiratory equipment and instilling saline into the child's tracheostomy on a regular basis. Chest physiotherapy and meticulous tracheo-bronchial toilet should also be performed on a regular basis, usually every 4 hr. These procedures may require increasing the delivered oxygen concentration to prevent hypoxia. Hyperinflation with air containing an increased amount of oxygen before and after suctioning can counteract the removal of oxygen from the airway. Stressful events that increase oxygen consumption and that may warrant a temporary increase in delivered oxygen concentration include chest physiotherapy, crying, and feeding.

Important nursing interventions include caring for the tracheostomy stoma and changing the cannula and securing it in place. Dressings at the tracheostomy site should be minimal. The cannula should be secured by methods that maximize the child's mobility safely. Clothing can be purchased or altered to allow clear visualization of the airway. The most common complications of artificial airways, obstruction, and accidental decannulation, can be prevented by using these measures.

Weaning: Nursing Assessment and Evaluation.   Weaning from respiratory support is influenced by developmental and family issues and is based on respiratory stability with a steady rate of weight gain and absence of intercurrent stress (Kettrick RG: unpublished abstract). It is a slow process, because the recovery from CRFI is slow. Weaning the child from support too rapidly increases susceptibility to infection and may worsen the respiratory failure. At The Children's Hospital of Philadelphia, recent studies of seven infants with CRFI due to BPD demonstrated that the mean age of weaning from support was 14.3 ± 3.5 months (range 12–22 months). During the 6–10-month age period a "turning point" occurred in which there was improvement in respiratory function accompanied by decreases in the PCO_2 and respiratory rate.[28] Increased weight gain was associated with this improvement.

Physical growth promotes the strengthening of diaphragmatic and accessory muscles and permits overall increased chest wall strength. Breaths become deeper and the respiratory rate decreases.[17] Concomitant with this decrease the work of breathing is diminished, and caloric expenditure can be used for growth. With continuing weight gain and developmental improvement the infant is able to tolerate lower levels of respiratory support.

Two approaches to weaning are generally considered. The first involves the gradual reduction in (1) the rate of intermittent mandatory ventilation (IMV), (2) the level of continuous positive airway pressure (CPAP), and (3) the concentration of inspired oxygen (FiO_2). The second approach allows gradual increases in periods of unassisted ventilation.[28] A level of respiratory support is provided with both approaches to maintain an $ETCO_2$ below 6.5% (PCO_2 approximately 45 to 50 torr) and a $TcPO_2$ from 60–90 torr.

With the first method of weaning, decreases in the rate of IMV are based on a respiratory rate below 60 breaths/min, absence of intercurrent stress, an $ETCO_2$ below 6.5%, a stable oxygenation status, a steady weight gain, and an appropriate activity level (Kettrick RG: unpublished abstract). Weans may occur each week or less frequently based on these variables. The criteria for CPAP weans are similar to those for IMV. Inspired oxygen concentration is decreased while the $TcPO_2$ is maintained between 60–90 torr. Stressful periods often require an increased concentration of inspired O_2 to achieve this value. When the end-point of weaning the child from CPAP and administered O_2 is approached, it is preferable to eliminate the CPAP first. CPAP equipment is cumbersome and stationary whereas portable O_2 equipment is compact, easy to manage, and allows the child to be mobile.

The second method of weaning may be considered with a toddler when mobility and activity are important developmental issues. Increased concentration of oxygen and, if necessary, CPAP are substituted for mandatory ventilation for short periods of time. Experience has revealed that, although this method of weaning is not preferable, it is acceptable and valuable in considering the child's total needs.

During the weaning process, evaluation of the adequacy of ventilation is based on weight, PO_2 and PCO_2 monitoring, and clinical observations. A chart for plotting weight, caloric intake, and changes in respiratory support can be useful in monitoring growth and response to weaning from support (Fig. 6.1).

Infection—Nursing Assessment and Intervention. The infant with CRFI is always at risk for intercurrent illness, such as pneumonia or acute bronchospasm.[28] Lung mechanics and overall strength and stamina determine responses to intercurrent stresses, including infection. All patients with tracheostomies have tracheal colonization with organisms not usually found in the tracheobronchial tree; it is a constant and expected occurrence. Tracheal colonization is characterized by the presence of two or three organisms in an amount less than 80%, as noted in cultures of tracheal aspirates. These organisms, which are usually gram-negative, become part of the child's normal flora. Consequently, the child will not show signs of infection. To avoid unnecessary treatment with antibiotics it is important to discriminate between tracheal colonization and infection. Complications of antibiotic therapy include renal toxicity, ototoxicity, and the development of antibiotic-resistant organisms.[25]

The child with CRFI may have recurrent respiratory infections. Tracheitis, bronchitis, and pneumonia occur most often with the organisms Pseudomonas

Fig. 6-1. Use of Weight, Caloric Intake, and Changes in Respiratory Support to Monitor Growth and Response to Weaning from Support.

Name: DK
Date of Birth: 5/5/81
Gestational Age: 27 weeks
Birth Weight: 900 gms.

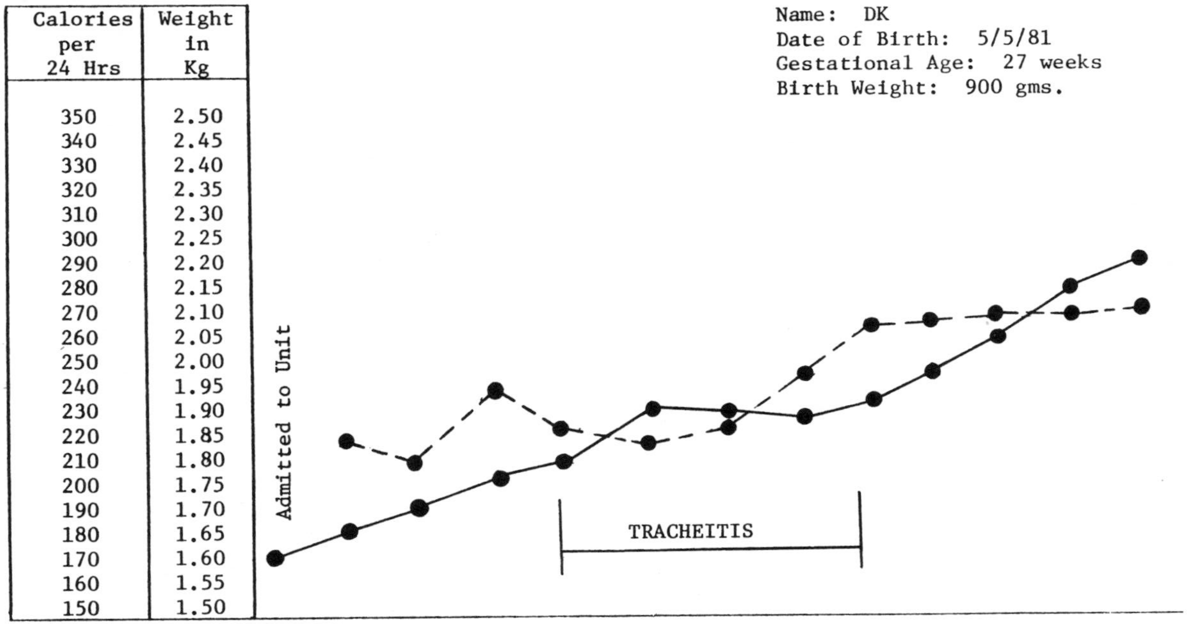

Calories per 24 Hrs	Weight in Kg
350	2.50
340	2.45
330	2.40
320	2.35
310	2.30
300	2.25
290	2.20
280	2.15
270	2.10
260	2.05
250	2.00
240	1.95
230	1.90
220	1.85
210	1.80
200	1.75
190	1.70
180	1.65
170	1.60
160	1.55
150	1.50

Legend:
Weight ——
Calories ----

Abbreviations:
IMV: Intermittent Mandatory Ventilation
FIO2: Fractional Inspired Oxygen
PEEP: Positive End Expiratory Pressure
IP: Inflating Pressure

	7/11	7/14	7/17	7/20	7/23	7/25	7/28	7/31	8/3	8/6	8/9	8/12	8/15
IMV	8.5	8.5	8.5	7.5	12	12	12	12	10	8.5	8.5	8.5	8.5
FIO2	.24	.24	.24	.24	.30	.30	.30	.30	.30	.30	.27	.27	.27
PEEP	8	8	8	8	8	8	8	8	8	8	8	7	7
IP	24	24	24	24	28	28	28	28	28	28	28	28	28

and Staphylococcus. Signs and symptoms of infection may include any or all of the following characteristics: a change in quantity, quality, or color of tracheal secretions; an increase in respiratory rate with retractions, flaring, and cyanosis; decreased appetite; increased gastric residuals; lethargy, irritability; fever; a culture of tracheal aspirate with greater than 80% of a pathogenic organism; and an increase in the white blood cell count (Kettrick RG: unpublished abstract). If cultures reveal multiple organisms without predominant flora, other manifestations of infection must be evaluated before making a decision to treat. An infection with a predominant flora (greater than 80%), an increased white blood cell count, and tracheal secretions that may plug and occlude the airway is treated with an antibiotic to which the infecting organism has demonstrated laboratory sensitivity. Infants who have been weaned on the basis of a stable respiratory status, a steady rate of growth, and an activity level appropiate for developmental progress are usually able to tolerate mild respiratory infections without an increase in support or worsening of the CRFI. Infections and other stresses, including operative procedures, may require temporary increases in support or a return to IMV. Such support conserves strength for the recovery process, avoids hypoxia and hypercarbia, and allows a return to maintenance support when the problem has been resolved.

Astute nursing observations can often detect infection before laboratory information becomes available or remarkable distress appears. Treatment with increased airway suctioning and chest physiotherapy can be initiated until laboratory information is available. Tracheal aspirates obtained weekly or more often for culture and sensitivity provide additional surveillance. Prevention of infection includes using aseptic technique with airway management (suctioning and tracheostomy cannula changes), strict handwashing between patient contacts, and changing equipment on a regular basis.

Altered Nutritional State

Providing nutritional support for the child with CRFI is a difficult and complex nursing problem. The child is subject to many stressors that hinder optimal growth. These may include (1) prematurity, (2) infections, (3) frequent surgical procedures, (4) cardiac and gastrointestinal anomalies, and (5) feeding dysfunctions. The weaning process and the growing child's activities of daily living increase his energy expenditure and caloric demand. Adequate nutrition is necessary to allow the child to develop strength, stamina, and improved pulmonary function with the growth of new lung tissue.[28] It also prevents immunologic compromise and decreases susceptibility to infection.

Nutritional management must deal with three basic concerns: (1) somatic growth is crucial for the growth of new lung tissue; (2) 120–200 Cal/kg/day are required for this growth to occur; and (3) feeding programs should maximize the developmental potential of the child.

The goals of the nurse include (1) formulating periodic nutritional assessments and evaluations; (2) providing adequate and appropriate intake; (3) monitoring diet tolerance, fluid status, and rate of growth; and (4) ameliorating and/ or preventing feeding dysfunctions.

Assessment. Anthropometric measurements are the best indicators of nutritional status. These include weight, height, head circumference, skin-fold thickness, and upper-arm circumference. The child with CRFI should be weighed on a regular basis, often daily. Daily weights also provide information about fluid balance. Length and head-circumference measurements are performed weekly. Consistent measurement by one person, possibly the primary nurse, is helpful to ensure accuracy. Triceps-skinfold thickness (TSF) indicates the amount of adipose tissue or of fat stores. The child with CRFI often has higher than normal fat stores related to his early and/or prolonged inactivity (Sandy Wilson, personal communication). As he becomes more active, an increase in muscle circumference occurs. The degree of skeletal muscle mass or protein stores is determined by measuring midarm muscle circumference.[29] Measurements of triceps skinfold thickness and arm muscle circumference may be obtained by the nurse or a nutrition consultant. Nutritional status is also assessed with laboratory measurements. Serum albumin and transferin concentrations are important indicators in determining protein requirements. The total lymphocyte count may be useful if malnutrition is suspected.[30]

Documenting intake for 24-hr periods and calculating the calories provide information on the quantity and quality of caloric intake. Weight, calories, and respiratory support can then be plotted on a growth chart (Fig. 6-1). Standardized growth charts can and should be used, but the nurse must consider the child's prematurity and plot according to the corrected gestational age. This adjustment should be used until 2-years of age (Sandy Wilson: personal communication).

Careful monitoring of the child's fluid and electrolyte status by the nurse is essential. Assessing fluid retention includes observing for the following signs and symptoms: sudden weight gain, decreased urinary output, puffy face, tachycardia, tachypnea, increased respiratory effort with retractions and nasal flaring, wheezing with râles heard on auscultation, cyanosis, high urine specific gravity, descending liver margin, and bulging fontanels in the young infant. Consistent observation of these parameters is vital because excessive fluid retention can severely compromise respiratory functioning.

Nursing Interventions. Providing adequate calories for growth and development is central to nutritional care. Determination of an appropriate diet should include considering several factors: the child's caloric requirements, his need for fluid restriction, the maximal protein recommendations, medications that inhibit nutrient absorption, and the renal solute load. The methods of feeding and the foods and textures that are offered to the child are equally important and may be the decisive factors in his taking in adequate amounts of food.

In determining the child's energy requirements, the nurse must consider his level of activity, stage of growth, and work of breathing. It is estimated that 45% of caloric intake for the infant is used for basal metabolism with 8–10% for new tissue growth and 38% for activity. Crying by itself can double the metabolic rate and require significant energy in even the most severely ill child.[31] Normal caloric requirements for growth for either gestational or chronologic age, are usually inadequate for the child with CRFI. In the first 6 months of life, the healthy infant requires 110–120 Cal/kg/day, whereas the premature infant requires 110–140 Cal/kg/day.[32] Caloric requirements also increase during the "catch-up" period in the premature infant. It is thought that this period of growth occurs at 8–10 months in girls and 6–8 months in boys. Therefore, caloric requirements for the child with CRFI may vary from 120–200 Cal/kg/day. A critical factor in determining the number of Cal/kg is the expenditure for the work of breathing. If the respiratory rate remains below 60 breaths/min, hypoxia and hypercarbia are absent as shown by non-invasive monitoring, and there are no clinical signs of respiratory distress, the energy expenditure for the work of breathing is considered acceptable. Calories are then available for growth. The child will also have energy to pursue developmental activities. Weight, linear growth, improvement in pulmonary function, and caloric requirements must be considered simultaneously, because increasing the intake to 200 Cal/kg/day may only result in deposition of excessive adipose tissue if pulmonary function and rate of linear growth are not considered.

Excessive fluid intake is often necessary to provide adequate caloric intake. Although the nurse can easily concentrate formula to increase calories without increasing fluid load, the renal solute load and the child's tolerance must be considered as well. Additional calories can be added through the use of high-calorie substances such as vegetable oil or glucose polymers. For the older child receiving tube feedings, commercially prepared feedings may be used along with vitamin supplementation. However, a blenderized mixture of a normal diet for age may be preferred to deliver essential amounts of nutrients.

The method of feeding, although based on the individual needs of each child, follows a fairly typical pattern. Enteral feedings are begun as soon as possible. The optimal progression is from continuous tube feedings to bolus feedings to oral feedings in the absence of an interruption in the gastrointestinal tract. The child with a permanent gastrostomy should progress to bolus feedings to increase his mobility and activity.

Feeding Dysfunction.   Similarly to the child's rate of growth, development of feeding behaviors is delayed, with both expected and uniquely associated problems. The development of feeding skills in normal infants occurs in a predictable sequence that is associated with the acquisition of function and behavior.[33] This sequence may not occur predictably in preterm infants. Premature infants usually have a weak suck and swallow. A functional swallow develops by 12.5 weeks of gestation and sucking behavior by 14 weeks, although coordination of these mechanisms does not occur until 32–34 weeks of gestational age.[32] Thus, the degree of prematurity and the severity of the child's illness influence his ability to experience normal feeding behaviors in the first weeks after birth.

The child who receives his nutritional support through intravenous and then tube feedings experiences inadequate oral stimulation.[34] As a result, behaviors that impede progression to oral feedings may develop. These aberrant behaviors include oral hypersensitivity, a hyperactive gag reflex, absent or ineffective sucking action, inadequate lip closure, tongue thrusting, and swallowing difficulties. Negative experiences with feeding may also contribute to behavioral difficulties. The child may have been "force-fed" in an effort to meet nutritional and caloric needs.[35] Another "negative" for the child is the often increased need for tracheal suctioning during feeding. Secretions increase in quantity during meals and interfere with breathing and swallowing when the child coughs in response to them. The child on a ventilator may also have abdominal distention, since more air is taken and swallowed during feeding. The increased volume of air needs to be expelled more frequently, and is often expelled forcefully and loudly; this may induce some vomiting. In addition, the child with CRFI may have associated neurologic problems or gastro-esophageal reflux that complicates feeding.

The nurse must use a variety of interventions to facilitate the development of feeding behavior. For children with oral hypersensitivity, a series of oral-digital stimulation exercises are often helpful.[34] This stimulation involves rubbing the child's shoulders, neck, cheeks, lips, gums, and tongue before each feeding to promote progressive desensitization. A hyperactive gag reflex often accompanies oral hypersensitivity. "Walking exercises," in which the nurse's fingertip is moved front-to-back on the child's tongue, can assist in desensitizing such a gag reflex. With all exercises, eliciting the gag response should be avoided as this reinforces undesirable behavior. Oral feedings should not be attempted until the hyperactive gag reflex has been diminished.

To facilitate the early acquisition of feeding behaviors and to prevent the troublesome problems of oral hypersensitivity and a hyperactive gag reflex, the use of pacifiers should always accompany tube feedings. The additional benefits of non-nutritive sucking include (1) development of muscles necessary for sucking and feedings; (2) development of a positive association between sucking and relief of hunger; and (3) initiation of the gastrointestinal cycle, thereby improving digestion.[35] All tube feedings should be preceeded by oral stimulation or by an attempt at bottle feeding when appropriate.

During both tube and bottle feedings, the child should be held and cuddled to develop a positive association between pleasure and the feeding experience. The child should be positioned in the nurse's arms with his head and hips flexed and his shoulders and arms in a forward position, with the arms brought to the midline and hyperextension of the head avoided.[33,34] This position facilitates the acquisition of more complex feeding skills.

When bottle-feeding the infant, the nurse should position her finger under the child's chin to enhance lip closure and to assist with sucking and swallowing. Oral feedings should take place with minimal distractions, with the nurse concentrating her total attention on the child and providing lavish praise as feeding skills are accomplished. Various textures, tastes, and colors of food provide new and interesting experiences for the child and enhance the progression of feeding behaviors.[32] As the child progresses to spoon and cup feedings, the use of a high chair for feeding will promote new behaviors. As he grows, every effort must be made to promote normal developmental progression by allowing and, indeed, encouraging the child to explore and experiment with his food. During this time of tasting and trying out new textures and uses of food, the nurse must carefully supervise the child to ensure his safety and the adequacy of this caloric intake.

Altered Sensory-Motor Development

Children with CRFI are particularly vulnerable to developmental delays and altered patterns of growth and development. Although it has been reported that ventilated infants with BPD do not differ in developmental outcome when matched with ventilated infants who did not experience BPD, follow-up studies of 10 survivors of prolonged mechanical ventilation report that half of the children were significantly delayed in achieving milestones.[5,16] Because of the heterogeneity of the population of children with CRFI, no one factor can be identified as the cause of the problem. The risk status of low-birth-weight infants has been well-documented.[36–40] The smaller the infant, the more vulnerable he seems to be, and it is the smallest, most immature infants who are likely to develop BPD. Fullterm infants who become ventilator-dependent because of congenital anomalies or perinatal mishaps are vulnerable to hypoxic episodes before or during mechanical ventilation. In both groups of infants, subsequent neurologic deficits may significantly impair development. Frequent episodes of acute illness, sensory overload, sleep deprivation, the lack of access to normal developmental experiences, immobilization, multiple caretakers, and separation from the home environment also contribute to delayed development.

It is vital that nurses caring for children with CRFI provide an environment that enhances the infant's ability to organize his behavior and his world and initiate a plan of care that provides periodic assessment of the infant's abilities and an individual program that supports continued development. Developmental care is based on the following principles:

1. The amount and quality of the interventions should be individualized based on the infant's state of development and recovery. Gestational age and perinatal morbidity are crucial variables in assessing infants and developing suitable programs.

2. Environmental events and stimuli have the potential to enhance the infant's ability to organize himself.

3. The environment should provide diurnal cycles and contingent responses to the infant.

4. The environment should facilitate and not violate the infant's biological rhythms.

5. Caregivers must view the infant holistically.[41]

The Nursing Environment. Guided by these principles, the nurse begins by carefully assessing the total ICU environment for stimuli or practices that may sabotage an infant's development. These include excessive noise,[42] a lack of diurnal rhythms, inconsistent patterns of patient assignment, unnecessary intrusions into the child's sleep–awake cycle for therapy or testing, and storage of equipment or placement of phones close to the child's bed. Interventions that create a more developmentally appropriate environment include arranging assignments to ensure that a relatively stable and small group of nurses care for the child, eliminating unnecessary noise, dimming the lights for naps and night sleeping, and providing a rhythm for each child's day. The nurse's ability to manipulate the environment is limited only by her creativity. She must develop skills in looking at the ICU with a "fresh eye" to identify and to modify creatively those elements that inhibit the infant's developmental progression.

Developmental Care of the Child.   The nurse also gathers data about the infant. A three-stage model for neurobehavioral development based on the work of Als and Brazelton is relevant for the infant with CRFI.[41] The nurse can use it as a basis for assessment and to plan interventions for the infant.

The three stages are integrity, "coming-out," and reciprocity. Integrity concerns the infant's physiologic organization. During this phase the infant must develop sufficient physical integrity and internal stability to use the caregiver's support and input for developmental gains. The infant whose heart rate decelerates with touching or position change is not ready for contingent stimulation. He cannot use it, and it is potentially dangerous.

When the baby is no longer critically ill, has achieved respiratory stability during mechanical ventilation, and can absorb enough calories for growth, he has reached the second, or "coming-out" phase. The infant in this stage is more alert in his response to outside stimuli. This is evident in his beginning attempts to suck and swallow his formula and by his "social" interest. It is during this phase that the caregiving environment can critically affect the physical well-being and growth of the high-risk infant. Each infant should be approached as an individual. Respect for the infant's sleep–wake cycle and feeding schedules must be incorporated into his care. Caregivers need to be sensitive to the infant's ability to cope with sensory stimulation. Some infants can tolerate the stimulation of one or two sensory modalities; others decompensate. During this stage, both positive and negative responses to caretaking activity may be expressed physiologically rather than interactively. Stressful experiences during feeding and caregiving can precipitate episodes of cyanosis and bradycardia. Conversely, autonomic nervous system organization is enhanced by sensitive care.

During the third stage of reciprocity, the developing relationship between the infant and caregiver plays a significant role in helping the infant to achieve active reciprocity with the social environment. Caretaking activities and sensory stimuli that are synchronized or contingent on the infant's behavior are essential. Noncontingent caretaking may disorganize the infant. Excessive noncontingent stimulation overloads the infant and causes him to withdraw. Measures that facilitate the infant's behavioral organization in this stage are swaddling, allowing the baby to discover and utilize his own self-quieting mechanisms, and using spontaneous alert periods for interactive play.[43]

As the child gets older and gains stamina, the nurse carefully structures the child's day to include normal developmental experiences such as brushing teeth and tub baths with water play. The child's parents should provide appropriate toys and clothing. Children must be "dressed for action" in age-appropriate clothes that have been modified to ensure easy access to the tracheostomy site. Clothing should allow unrestricted movement and be suitable for the day's play and feeding activities. Play is the "work of childhood" and children with CRFI should have regularly scheduled periods of play out of bed. Indeed, as the child's age increases, the majority of his daytime should be spent in play activities outside of the crib. A play therapist is an integral part of developmental care. The therapist directly interacts with the child during activities such as dancing and "making" music and provides valuable play ideas to both nurses and parents. Mats, "jolly-jumpers," rocking horses, scooter cars, and walkers are useful to encourage gross motor activities. Respiratory equipment can be modified to increase the length of ventilator tubing and the distance from sources of compressed air and oxygen to permit a wider range of exploration by the child. (These modifications should be initiated only after consultation with the physician managing the child's respiratory care and with the respiratory therapist.) With increased stamina the child may be able to tolerate short periods of time off the ventilator. These periods should be used for excursions outside the unit to a planned physical therapy program or to places of interest in the hospital (i.e., fountains, fish tanks, snack bar, picnic area). Parents who have learned to care for the child's special respiratory needs can use these trips as private times with their child.

Regularly scheduled nap times are part of the rhythm of the child's day. Because the child with CRFI has usually been nursed on his back for the first several months of his life, his shoulders are retracted, neck and back are extended, and hips are abducted. This positioning may contribute to delayed development unless remedial action is taken. The child should be placed in a prone or side-lying position during naps. The former position encourages the use of arm extensor muscles; the latter position promotes symmetrical development, brings hands to the midline, and prevents permanent hip abduction. These behaviors are essential if the child is to learn to sit and crawl.

As the child increases in cognitive and motor abilities, limit setting becomes an important aspect of care that is necessary to ensure the child's personal safety and to promote the acquisition of socially desirable behaviors. The ventilator-dependent child, like all children, loves to explore his surroundings. His environment differs from that of other children in that it includes EKG leads, ventilator tubing and alarms, and a tracheostomy tube. He soon learns the attention-getting value of exploring the machinery that is so much a part of his life, and the initial exploratory behavior evolves into a potentially life-threatening game. Setting limits is an integral, though difficult part of care. Parents and nurses must collaborate in deciding the methods of discipline to be used, since consistency is fundamental to the success of any method. They must agree on the behaviors to be reinforced, those that will be ignored, and those for which the child will be disciplined. Disciplinary measures include using a stern voice, expressing verbal disapproval, avoiding eye contact with the child, using an expressionless face, stopping play activities, and—lastly— isolating the child in the crib with the curtains drawn and monitor alarms intact and functioning. Physical punishment should never be used.

Another important developmental area of concern is the child's acquisition of speech and language. In the child with CRFI such acquisition may be delayed or prevented because of the following factors: (1) dependence on ventilatory support, (2) impaired integrity of the upper airway, (3) absence of oral stimulation and feeding experiences, (4) hearing impairment (either congenital or acquired), and (5) environmental impediments.[34] The ventilator-dependent child may learn to vocalize while receiving high inspiratory pressures. A leak of air around the tracheostomy cannula may allow air to pass upward and over the vocal chords during inspiration.[34] However, as the child is weaned, this method of speech is dysfunctional, because he must learn to vocalize with expiration. Therefore, the total communication approach that uses sign language, speech, and other forms of communication is an integral part of development care. The nurse, assisted by a speech pathologist, must coordinate a functional communication system for the child.

The infant with CRFI expresses his needs through normal patterns of crying or smiling although vocalizations usually do not occur with the crying. The child may progress to using clicking and kissing sounds or buccal speech to gain attention and to communicate.[34,44] As the child grows, a system to communicate needs to ease frustration can be developed. Sign language or the use of gestures has been found most effective. The child often first learns signs that apply to daily needs (e.g., tracheal suctioning or a diaper change) and then moves to more complex gestures. All professionals interacting with the child must be provided with continuing education to provide consistency in communicating with the child. The nurse should speak as she signs in an effort to encourage the child to imitate mouth movements. With this structured program the use of sign language gradually diminishes and disappears as vocalization becomes possible.[34] When appropriate, alternate means of communication including esophageal speech and sign boards may be used. The nurse must remember that communication is important to other developmental activities. Her stimulation via talking to the child and explaining activities is as important in developmental intervention as the activities themselves.

An adjunct to care is a formal program of developmental assessment and intervention. The Portage Guide to Early Education is one such program.[45] The program has three parts: a direction manual, a check-list of behaviors used for assessing the child's developmental progress, and a card file listing specific interventions that promote development. The Portage Guide differs from infant stimulation programs in that it assesses behavior and suggests intervention in five different areas (socialization, language, cognition, self-help, and motor activities) until the developmental age of 6 years. This makes it especially useful for infants with CRFI who may be hospitalized for 1–3 years. It is also an excellent tool for encouraging parental collaboration because of its simplicity and emphasis on mastering milestones. Parents and nurses can work together to discover the skills that the child has mastered and decide after consulting the checklist which behaviors are to be encouraged in the developmental care plan. Not only are both parents and nurses motivated to carry out the mutually agreed on plan, but also the checklist reminds them of the child's progress. A drawback of the Guide is that is was developed for healthy children and does not delineate problems with enough precision in ventilator-dependent children. The use of the guide must be accompanied by an on-going assessment that describes the quality of the mastery of milestones and by a program of physical and occupational therapy if the child's maximum developmental potential is to be achieved.

Altered Family Relationships

Families at Risk   The events that occur around the time of an infant's birth, the attitudes and ideas of primary caregivers, and the quality of the early environment have a profound effect on a family's development and on establishing interpersonal relationships within the family. The earliest experience of family life for families of children with CRFI occur within the milieu of the IICU. Although elements of this type of experience are shared with parents of other sick or premature infants, the experience taken as a whole is unique because—rather than lasting a few days or weeks—it often extends into months and years before a positive outcome is achieved. To compound the problem further, children with CRFI are part of a well-recognized and well-documented population of children at risk for family dysfunction: premature infants, those with congenital anomalies, and those who are chronically ill. The long-term nature of CRFI, coupled with the high-risk status of the children, challenges parents and nurses to work together creatively to ensure optimal family functioning in what is, at best, a most peculiar situation.

The birth of a premature or sick infant places unusual demands on a family. If the child develops CRFI, the problem, with its chronic nature interspersed with frequent periods of crisis, may keep the family in a prolonged period of disorganization and uncertainty. The parents' first task is to work through their grief, because their initial pervasive feeling is one of loss. The expected healthy infant is replaced by a seriously ill "high-risk" infant. This underreactive infant replaces the responsive infant with whom the parents has expected to interact actively. Separation replaces the anticipated close contact. A warmer bed in an IICU replaces the bassinette beside the mother's bed. The parents are displaced as the primary caregivers by doctors and nurses. The mother, in particular, rather than gaining self-esteem and success in parenthood, perceives herself as a failure.[46] If the infant has been born prematurely, the mother has not experienced the achievement of her final tasks of pregnancy, the cognitive and emotional preparation for labor and delivery, and the readiness to assume a caretaking relationship with her child. Labor and delivery have been unexpected and frightening experiences for her. She may not be ready to parent the infant. This is manifested cognitively by her feeling that she cannot believe that the baby is hers and practically by the lack of concrete preparation for the baby, such as the purchasing of a crib or infants' clothing (Schraeder BD; unpublished Master's Thesis). These experiences are mingled with intense grieving characterized by anger, loss of appetite, guilt, sadness, disbelief, depression, crying, and praying for the infant's recovery.[47] As the weeks go on, coping patterns are established, but the anxiety and grief, often just below the surface, may reappear at various times during the course of the child's hospitalization. Acute illnesses or set-backs in the child's recovery, important events like Christmas or a birthday that are celebrated in the ICU, or a friend's delivery of a healthy new baby, can precipitate renewed feelings of sadness. Providing a forum to express this grief and creating an environment that nurtures hope are integral parts of sensitive nursing care.

In addition to resolving their loss and establishing adaptive coping mechanisms, parents must learn to love and care for this "new" infant who has replaced their expected healthy infant. There is evidence that parents of children with congenital anomalies and parents of premature infants experience difficulty in negotiating this task.[48] Children who are born prematurely are over-represented in studies of abused and neglected children.[49]

For the child with CRFI, the family concerns usually associated with prematurity are aggravated by the extreme separation and despair characteristic of long-term hospitalization. Parents are overwhelmed by the complexity of the child's physical problems and his dependence on technology for survival. They often cope with their feelings by avoiding the child and/or adopting a parenting style that focuses exclusively on the pathophysiology or technology associated with the child's disease. The result of both coping strategies is the failure to relate to the "real" baby—through either sporadic, inconsistent visiting and calling patterns or overintellectualization of his problems.

Avoiding or minimalizing dysfunctional coping styles depends on recognizing the risk and identifying potential problems at an early stage. All families of children with CRFI experience an altered parent-child relationship. It is imperative that the nurse recognize this problem and accord it the same degree of concern and professional involvement that characterizes the treatment of physiologically-based problems. Parents must become partners in the child's care if there is to be a positive outcome. In addition to nurturing hope and assisting parents to deal with their grief, nurses must create an environment that fosters the growth of parental love and family commitment to the infant. This goal is accomplished through the use of the nursing process based on a conceptual framework.

Conceptual Parenting Model and Nursing Process. A model of parenting based on Riva Rubins' theory of "binding-in" is an effective conceptual base for working with parents of children with CRFI.[50] The development of parenting is placed on a continuum that begins with a "getting-acquainted" or touching stage, continues through the establishment of a caretaking relationship with the infant, and finally progresses to an identity stage. During this last phase, the child is incorporated into the family. Although elements of each stage may overlap, nursing assessment, diagnosis, intervention, and evaluation are based on parental behaviors and cues.

Assessment.   Assessment includes the gathering of both subjective and objective data. Because this is a family-based model, data must be gathered on the components of the family system. An efficient and useful tool is a family genogram[51], very similar to the one used to construct a family medical history. The important element of this genogram is not the family history of disease but the identification of variables that are important which contribute to a family's strengths and limitations. The genogram yields data on family educational level, ethnicity, socio-economic status, the ages and genders of immediate and extended family members, number of siblings, and information concerning important events in the family's history: dates of marriages, divorces, non-legal but important alliances, births, and deaths. It is useful for two reasons: it reinforces for both nurses and parents the notion that the family is the unit of care and provides information that is valuable to structure interventions—for instance, mobilizing family support systems, providing child care for children at home while the parents are visiting, and identifying sources of support if homecare is considered.

The nurse also gathers objective data on the parents' stage of grieving and their use of coping strategies. Finally, data is gathered on the parents' relationship with the child and their stage of parenting. This is accomplished principally by listening for verbal cues and observing behaviors.

Goals of Care and Intervention Strategies.   Goals are based on the assessment data and are derived from the nursing diagnosis of altered parent–child relationships. The nurse analyzes behavioral and objective data and places the parents into the appropriate stages of parenting behavior (touching, caretaking, and identifying). For instance, a parent who stands by a child's crib or isolette, staring at the child or venturing to touch him with the finger tips only when urged by the nurse, and whose questions and observations focus exclusively on the equipment or the child's "numbers" is in the very initial stage of parenting. An appropriate nursing goal at that stage is the parent's spontaneous demonstration of early parenting behaviors: whole-hand touching, stroking, and holding the infant in "en face" position. Nursing interventions should enhance opportunities for these behaviors and refocus the parent on the "baby" qualities of the infant. Parents in IICUs learn to parent their infant by watching the way in which nurses interact with the child; therefore specific nursing interventions must include role modeling. Nurturing behaviors, stroking, talking, and gentle handling convey to parents that this is a baby, not simply an "artifact of medical technology." Other ways of reinforcing this concept are providing spontaneous personalized information about the infant and responding to questions about the child's physical state. Nurses, often without realizing it, are expert observers of their patient's state, levels of behavioral organization, and growth and development. The nurse must share this information, because it provides parents with a dimension of reality that is difficult to perceive in an infant who is invaded and supported by tubes and machinery.

Table 6-1 Stages of Parenting Behaviors and Nursing Interventions*

Parenting Behavior	Nursing Interventions

Stage I: Touching
  Uses fingertips
  Uses whole hand
  Strokes child
  Holds and studies child "en face"
  Spontaneously lowers crib rails to fondle, hold, or talk to child.
	Establish trust between the nurse and the parents
	Teach parents their parental rights and responsibilities
	Establish patterns of communication between staff and parents
	Assist parents to hold child comfortably
	Serve as role model for nurturing behaviors
	Identify infant competencies, behavioral style, preferences
	Involve parents in formulating plan for infant's stimulation care plan

Stage II: Care-taking
  Provides clean clothing, toys, grooming aids
  Performs activities of daily living (bathing, diapering, feeding, dressing)
  Performs care-taking tasks with proficiency and expresses pleasure in meeting infant's needs
  Comforts child when he is distressed or crying
  Meets child's special health needs (suctioning, cleaning stoma sites, treatments)
	Develop and implement teaching plans for parents
	Continue to assist parents to "know" their baby
	Provide information on infant growth and development
	Support parents' newly-learned skills

Stage III: Identity
  Brings linens from home
  Takes photographs
  Brings individualized toys
  Makes personalized observations about child
  Offers suggestions and makes demands for personalized care
  Demonstrates "advocacy" behavior
  Feels he/she can care for child better than anyone else
  Demonstrates consistent visiting and/or calling pattern
  Focuses questions on total child, not only on physiologic parameters
	Show sensitivity to role of parents
	Accept parents' need for privacy (both psychologic and physical) with the infant
	Encourage parental actions indicating that the child has been incorporated into the family; e.g.; parent's providing linens, clothing, grooming aides and toys from home
	Encourage visits by siblings, extended family and/or significant others
	Teach and support parents' advocacy on behalf of their child

Evaluation. The evaluation and revision of goals is a continuous process. Evaluation criteria are based on observable, patient-centered goals. The nurse formulates new goals based on the Rubin's model and develops new intervention strategies utilizing the individual parents' strengths and limitations.

During the second stage, parents achieve proficiency and pleasure in caring for their baby. This includes for a child with CRFI, learning to bathe, feed and dress an infant who has a tracheostomy and ventilator tubing, and to suction the airway and change tracheostomy strings. Postponing the teaching of these skills until the time of discharge prevents parents from truly feeling comfortable with their child. The machinery and tubes remain a mystery to them and may present a barrier to "knowing" him. Once comfortable with the skills necessary to meet the child's special needs, parents are confident and have the courage to pull the curtains around the crib, or turn their backs to a busy ICU and enjoy a private time with their child.

Parents may then move to the third stage of parenting—identity. During this stage, they incorporate the child into their family. He has become an integral part of the family unit in spite of his physical separation from their home. They freely excercise their rights and responsibilities as parents.

The accompanying chart (Table 6-1) more fully describes the parenting stages and appropriate nursing interventions. It is designed as a guide, not a rigid formula. The nursing process should be implemented on an individualized basis, as a product of the creative interaction between the nurse and the family.

THE NURSING ROLE IN CARING FOR THE VENTILATOR-DEPENDENT CHILD

The provision of high-quality, long-term nursing care in a system intended for acute short-term management presents a special challenge to critical care nurses. All of the systems are designed to serve a very different patient population from the child needing chronic care. Physicians may rotate on and off the service on a monthly basis; visiting may be restricted to parents; charts are set up for hour-to-hour assessments and are irrelevant and inappropriate for the child whose admission may last 1–2 years. In ICUs safety and vigilance take precedence over developmental or affective needs. The nurse must use her skills as an innovator to develop new systems and standards of care for the child with CRFI that do not compromise quality.

Another challenge of long-term care is the nature of the relationship between the nurse, the infant, and the family. The long-term contact, the frequent crises, and the shared celebration of important events usually restricted to family members, generates in the nurse feelings of love and commitment to the child and his family. This devotion can have a positive effect; indeed, the child needs loving, as well as skilled caregivers to grow and to thrive. But the creative use of this emotional investment in an environment that values objective data, technical competence and "coolness" challenges everyone involved with the child's care.[52–54] To manage successfully the roles of innovator and "significant other", the nurse must have insight into her own inner strengths and limitations and must utilize a care delivery system that maximizes her professional potential.

Primary nursing is an integral part of the care given to ventilator-dependent children and their parents.[50] The primary nurse—in collaboration with four or five permanent nursing team members—plans, implements, and coordinates care. She establishes a therapeutic relationship with the child and his family.

This relationship is based on trust and open communication. The primary nurse is responsible for the child's nursing care on a 24-hr a day basis and has the authority to represent the nursing staff at interdisciplinary meetings. Care must be taken when assigning a particular nurse to a family, for it is an awesome responsibility. The decision must be a thoughtful one based on the child's needs and the nurses' strengths.[55] The nurse must possess superb communication skills; the confidence, tact, and poise to collaborate successfully with other disciplines; and the maturity to work with families and children in a situation where the outcome is uncertain. She must be sensitive to the child's developmental needs and possess the knowledge base and the creativity to enhance developmental opportunities. Because the nurse–patient relationship may last for many months or years, it is difficult, and perhaps, impossible for the nurse to maintain total objectivity about the patient and his family. It has been suggested that nurses who provide care for chronically ill children often assume the role of "significant other." Significant others value the child and may even love the child. They learn to cope with the child's chronic illness by "building up their functions within the situation while at the same time scaling down expectations of one's self."[56] An effective primary nurse understands that despite the giving of herself, her energies, and her hopes, she cannot change the nature of the problem. She can, however, support hope and provide a decent quality of life for children and their parents.

An essential component and built-in strength of primary nursing with patient-determined nursing care teams is the opportunity for peer support and review. Collegial relationships characterized by interdependence and trust offer support for nurses caring for children whose long-term illnesses are characterized by frequent set-backs and crises. The support is strengthened by a head nurse who is an empathic listener, teacher, and counselor to the primary nurses and other members of the nursing care teams. The head nurse is responsible for developing in the staff the affective, cognitive, and psychomotor dimensions necessary for the provision of care to the child with CRFI. These include

1. Fostering a caring attitude that recognizes the inherent worth and dignity of the individual
2. Fostering the belief that nurses have the ability and the responsibility to improve the quality of life
3. Providing opportunities for the staff to improve its communication and collaborative skills
4. Supporting the provision of family-centered nursing care
5. Assisting the staff to increase its knowledge to provide developmental nursing care.
6. Urging the staff to incorporate the principles and skills of rehabilitative nursing into practice

Another source of valuable support to the nursing staff and other members of the health care team is the psychiatric liaison. This individual, often a psychiatrist or psychiatric nurse, may meet with the staff at periodic, regularly scheduled intervals or when specific problems or crises arise. It is important that this individual is a "part of" but not "from" the critical care staff. He or she must be close enough to understand the pressures and issues but distanced enough to possess a fresh perspective. Used effectively, the liaison can offer valuable insight, help focus a problem or issue, or simply provide a sounding board for the necessary airing of insolvable problems.

Research and Future Directions

The current published research on CRFI is sparse and is concerned with describing the nature of the phenomenon. This research, which has been conducted exclusively by medical practitioners, has focused on pulmonary function,[16,17] correlations between physical growth and successful weaning,[37] and patient outcome.[5] These studies, though flawed by small sample size and limited follow-up, have yielded valuable information on the relationship between somatic growth and pulmonary function and on the efficacy of a program of prolonged weaning. These studies also suggest that families can view the experience of prolonged and intensive support for their children from a positive perspective and that CRFI does not always result in significant development delay.[5] These issues need more study by a multi-disciplinary research team using a larger sample size, standardized tools for measuring family well-being and developmental outcome of the child, and a longitudinal design. Another area of research is to determine the effects of care when children with CRFI are cared for in one of three settings: the ICU, a specialty unit for ventilator-dependent children, or the home. An important nursing research problem is to compare outcomes between children whose parents visit consistently and those who are visited sporadically.

No discussion of future directions in the care of CRFI is complete without emphasis on the most important aspect—its prevention. The keystone of prevention is better maternal nutrition, optimal spacing of pregnancies, genetic counseling and early identification of high-risk mothers, and their management in perinatal centers capable of providing continuous care from conception to discharge of mother and baby from the hospital. It has been estimated that in 60–75% of the cases, the sick neonate was a distressed fetus whose vulnerability could have been identified during the mother's pregnancy.[57] Nurses in critical care settings must broaden their practice to include an interest and involvement in preventive measures. On a national and community level, this means supporting programs that are designed to improve the reproductive outcome of mothers and infants. Professionally, critical care nurses must involve themselves in consumer education and must support efforts to regionalize and centralize perinatal care.

In presenting the care of the child with CRFI we have tried to stress the positive impact of the experience, the emotional maturity that occurs from weathering adversity, the potential for the growth of love and commitment, and the confidence that comes from successful rehabilitation to both caregivers and recipients. But the human and material toll is enormous. The monetary expenditures can be measured, but the human expenditures are incalculable.[58]

The future directions of care lie very clearly in prevention. Until that time, nurses who practice in critical care settings must strive to improve the quality of life of the children and families in their care and must support efforts to identify and maximize programs that contribute to reproductive health.

REFERENCES

1. Edwards DD, Dyer WW, Northway WH: Twelve years experience with bronchopulmonary dysplasia. Pediatrics 59:839, 1977
2. Stocks J, Godfrey S: The role of artificial ventilation, O_2, and CPAP in the pathogenesis of lung damage in neonates: assessments by serial measurements of lung function. Pediatrics 57:352, 1976
3. Taghizadeh A, Reynolds EOR: Pathogenesis of bronchopulmonary dysplasia following hyaline membrane disease. Am J Pathol 82:241, 1976
4. Watts J, Ariagno R, Brady J: Chronic pulmonary disease in neonates after artificial ventilation: distribution of ventilation and pulmonary interstitial emphysema. Pediatrics 60:273, 1977
5. Ziegler M, Shaw S, Goldberg A, Kettrick R, Koop CE: Sequelae of prolonged ventilatory support for pediatric surgical patients. Pediatr Surg 14(6):768–772, 1979
6. Kettrick R: Chronic respiratory failure in infancy. Lecture presented at Pediatric Anesthesia and Critical Care, The Children's Hospital of Philadelphia, April 2–6, 1979 (abstract–unpublished)
7. Schraeder B: A creative approach to caring for the ventilator dependent child. Am J Matern Child Nurs 4:165, 1979
8. Kattan M: Long-term sequelae of respiratory illness in infancy and childhood. Pediatr Clin North Am 26:525, 1979
9. Cox JM: Prolonged pediatric ventilatory assistance and related problems. Crit Care Med 1:158, 1973
10. Northway W, Rosan RC, Porter D: Pulmonary disease following respiratory therapy of hyaline-membrane disease. N Engl J Med 276:357, 1967
11. Northway W: Observations on bronchopulmonary dysplasia. J Pediatr 95:815, 1979
12. Fitzhardinge PM: Follow-up studies in infants treated by mechanical ventilation. Clin Perinatol 5:451, 1978
13. Stahlman MT: Clinical description of bronchopulmonary dysplasia. J Pediatr 95:829, 1979
14. Bancolari E, Abdenour GE, Feller R, Gannon J: Bronchopulmonary dysplasia: clinical presentation. J Pediatr 5:819, 1979
15. Downes JJ: Long-term respiratory support of infants. Paper presented at the University of Utah Perinatal/Pediatric Anesthesia Symposium, Salt Lake City, Utah, February 19, 1978
16. Loeber NV, Morray J, Kettrick R, Downes J: Pulmonary function in chronic respiratory failure of infancy. Crit Care Med 8:597, 1980
17. Morray JP, Fox WW, Swedlow DB, et al.: Pulmonary function in bronchopulmonary dysplasia. Crit Care Med 8:228, 1980
18. Pinney P, Cotton EK: Home management of bronchopulmonary dysplasia. Pediatrics 58:856, 1976
19. Moylar F, O'Connel K, Todres D, Shannon DC: Edema of the pulmonary interstitium in infants and children. Pediatrics 55:783, 1975

20. Fox WW: Bronchopulmonary dysplasia (respirator lung syndrome): clinical course and outpatient therapy. Pediatr Ann 7:40, 1978
21. Rooklin AR, Moomjian AS, Shutak JG, et al.: Theophylline therapy in bronchopulmonary dysplasia. J Pediatr 95:882, 1979
22. Patterson RH, Gustafson EA, Sheridan E: Falconer's Current Drug Handbook 1980–82. Philadelphia, WB Saunders, 1980
23. Huang N: The use of new antibiotic agents for chronic pulmonary disease. Pediat Ann 7:28, 1979
24. Morray JP, Fox WW, Kettrick RG, Downes JJ: Improvement in lung mechanics as a function of age in the infant with severe bronchopulmonary dysplasia. Pediatr Res (In press), 1981
25. Finer NN: Newer trends in continuous monitoring of critically ill infants and children. Pediatr Clin North Am 27:553, 1980
26. Huch A, Huch R: Transcutaneous non-invasive monitoring of PO_2. Hosp Pract 11:43–52, 1976
27. Fisher DM, Swedlow DB: Estimating $PaCO_2$ by end-tidal gas sampling in children. Crit Care Med 9:287, 1981
28. Morray JP, Fox WW, Kettrick RG, Downes JJ: Clinical correlates of successful weaning in severe bronchopulmonary dysplasia. Crit Care Med 9(12):815, 1981
29. Pollack M, Wiley J, Holbrook P: Early nutritional depletion in critically ill children. Crit Care Med 9:580, 1981
30. Reimer S, Michener W, Steiger E: Nutritional support of the critically ill child. Pediatr Clin North Am 27:647, 1980
31. Czajka-Narins D, Weil W: Calories. In: Developmental Nutrition. eds. Oliver K, Ross Laboratories: 9, 1979
32. Whaley L, Wong D: Nursing Care of Infants and Children. St. Louis, CV Mosby, 1979
33. Pipes P: Nutrition in Infancy and Childhood. St Louis, CV Mosby, 1981
34. Simon B, Handler SD: The speech pathologist and management of children with tracheostomies. J Otolaryngol 10(6):440, 1981
35. Measel CP, Anderson GC: Non-nutritive sucking during tube feedings: effect on clinical course in premature infants. JOGN 8(5):265, 1979
36. Boyle M, Giffen A, Fitzhardinge P: The very low birthweight infant: impact on parents during the pre-school years. Early Hum Dev 1:191, 1977
37. Bhat R, Raju T, Vidyasagar D: Immediate and long-term outcome of infants less than 1,000 grams. Crit Care Med 6:147, 1978
38. Lubchenco LD, Delivoria-Papadopoulos M, Butterfield L et al.: Long-term follow-up studies of prematurely born infants. I. Relationship of handicaps to nursery routines. J Pediatr 80:501, 1972
39. Lubchenco L, Delivoria-Papadopoulos M, Searls D: Long-term follow-up studies of prematurely born infants. II. Influence of birth weight and gestational age on sequelae. J Pediatr 80:509, 1972
40. Rubin R, Rosenblatt C, Balow B: Psychological and educational sequelae of prematurity. Pediatrics 52:352, 1973
41. Als H, Lester BM, Brazelton TB: Dynamics of the behavioral organization of the premature infant: a theoretical perspective. In: Infants Born at Risk. eds. Field T New York, SP Med and Scientific Books, 1979
42. Lawson K, Daum C, Turkowitz J: Environmental characteristics of a neonatal intensive-care unit. Child Dev 48:1633, 1977

43. Gorski P, Davison M, Brazelton TB: Stages of behavioral organization in the high-risk neonate: theoretical and clinical considerations. Semin Perinatol 3:61, 1979

44. Kaslon KW, Grabo DE, Rubin RT: Voice, speech, and language habilitation in young children without laryngeal function. Arch Otolaryngol 104:737, 1978

45. Portage Guide to Early Education, Portage, W. Available from Cooperative Educational Service Agency 12, 412 East Slifer Street, Portage, WI 53901

46. Taylor P, Hall B: Parent-infant bonding: problems and opportunities in a perinatal center. Semin Perinatol 3:73, 1979

47. Benfield DG, Leib SA, Rulter J: Grief response of parents after referral of the cricially ill newborn to a regional center. N Engl J Med 294:975, 1976

48. McCormick MC, Shapiro S, Starfield BH: Rehospitalization in the first year of life for high-risk survivors. Pediatrics 66:991, 1980

49. Klein M, Stern L: Low birth weight and the battered child syndrome. Am J Dis Child 122:15, 1971

50. Schraeder BD: Attachment and parenting despite lengthy intensive care MCN, 5:37, 1980

51. Hurley PM: Family assessment: systems theory and the genogram. Children's Health Care J. of the Assoc. for the Care of Children's Health 10(3):76–82, 1982

52. Consalva C: Nurse turnover in the newborn intensive care unit. JOGN Nurs 8:201, 1979

53. Jacobson S: Stressful situations for neonatal intensive care nurses. MCN, 3:144, 1978

54. Marshall R, Kuzman G: Burnout in the neonatal intensive care unit. Pediatrics 65(6):1161–1165, 1980

55. Ciske K: Accountability: the essence of primary nursing. Am J Nurs 79:891, 1979

56. Steele S: A holistic approach to coping with health impairment. Paper presented at 2nd Annual National Pediatric Nursing Conference, Philadelphia, 1977

57. Korones S: High-risk Newborn Infants. St. Louis, CV Mosby Company, 1981

58. Butnaresque G: Prenatal Nursing. New York, John Wiley and Sons, 1980

7 Congenital Heart Disease: Critical Perioperative Nursing Management

Margaret C. Slota
Lee B. Beerman

Approximately 8 of every 1000 children born in this country have some form of congenital heart disease. In many of these children the heart defect is mild and will never require catheterization, surgery, or even significant restriction of activity. However, in approximately one of six affected children the cardiac anomaly is severe enough to require surgery within the 1st year of life. Thus, over 5000 infants under 1 year of age and thousands more older children will undergo cardiac surgery each year.[1]

In the last decade tremendous strides have been made in the technical abilities of cardiac surgeons to physiologically correct or to palliate almost all forms of congenital heart disease. Advances in intraoperative techniques, such as profound hypothermia, circulatory arrest or low-flow cardiopulmonary bypass, and myocardial preservation have obviously been crucial in the progress that has been made. However, improved and more sophisticated perioperative care has been just as important in the remarkably improved survival of critically ill infants and children undergoing heart surgery.

In this chapter, we will discuss a general approach to the types of congenital defects that most commonly require surgical intervention, currently used intraoperative techniques, and considerations of postoperative management.

DEFECTS REQUIRING SURGERY: IMPLICATIONS FOR PERIOPERATIVE MANAGEMENT

The number and complexity of possible congenital heart defects can be bewildering unless a simplified classification scheme is used. The most common approach (Table 7-1) is based on whether cyanosis is present and whether pulmonary blood flow is decreased, normal, or increased.

Acyanotic Lesions With Increased Pulmonary Blood Flow

Included in the category of acyanotic lesions with increased pulmonary blood flow (i.e., classic left-to-right shunts) is the ventricular septal defect (VSD), the congenital anomaly that is most likely to require surgery. Endocardial cushion defect (ECD) is the most commonly occurring defect in children with Down's syndrome. Other frequently seen lesions in this category are patent ductus arteriosus (PDA) and atrial septal defect (ASD).

Depending on severity, these lesions share to varying degrees the physiologic consequences of a large left-to-right shunt: volume overload with chronic congestive heart failure, pulmonary hypertension with or without elevated pulmonary vascular resistance, malnutrition and failure to thrive, and pulmonary parenchymal disease. Pre- and postoperative implications are discussed below.

Congestive Heart Failure (CHF).   CHF that is unresponsive to medical management is probably the most common indication for surgery for VSD or ECD. If the clinical findings of tachypnea, labored respirations, tachycardia, hepatomegaly, and feeding difficulties persist in spite of an adequate trial of digitalis and diuretics, little is gained by delaying surgical intervention. Any child with significant CHF prior to surgery can be expected to have some degree of myocardial depression postoperatively. Therefore, digitalis therapy and intermittently administered diuretics are generally required after the patient returns from surgery to the ICU. Further support of myocardial pump function

Table 7-1. Classification of Congenital Heart Disease

Acyanotic	
Increased pulmonary blood flow	Normal pulmonary blood flow
Ventricular septal defect (VSD)	Aortic valvular stenosis (ASV)
Atrial septal defect (ASD)	Pulmonic valvular stenosis (PSV)
Patent ductus arteriosus (PDA)	Coarctation of the aorta (COA)
Endocardial cushion defect (ECD)	

Cyanotic	
Decreased pulmonary blood flow	Normal or increased pulmonary blood flow
Tricuspid atresia (TAT)	Transposition of the great arteries (TGA)
Tetrology of fallot (TOF)	Total anomalous pulmonary venous return
Pulmonary atresia (PAT)	(TAPVR)
Critical pulmonic stenosis (CPS)	Truncus arteriosus (TRU)

with catecholamine therapy such as dopamine (Intropin) is also frequently needed for a period of time. These comments apply to both open-heart corrective procedures and palliative operations (i.e., pulmonary banding). In the former case, cardiopulmonary bypass and/or ventriculotomy can lead to further myocardial depression, which may be temporary or prolonged. In the case of pulmonary banding, inadequate reduction of pulmonary blood flow related to a loose band may result in persistent heart failure. Another difficulty in the perioperative management of these patients is often manifested in the operating room. In an effort to maximize control of the symptoms of CHF, diuretics are sometimes administered excessively, resulting in significant volume contraction. The infant may appear to be relatively stable, but during induction of anesthesia an episode of severe hypotension and/or cardiorespiratory arrest may occur. This occurrence is caused by vasodilatation secondary to the anesthetic agent accompanied by a critical reduction of filling pressures (i.e., left and right atrial pressures) to levels inadequate for ventricular function.

Pulmonary Hypertension.   This complication most commonly results from a large VSD or an ECD. The rate at which the pulmonary hypertension and pulmonary vascular disease progress is extremely variable, but it is very unusual for irreversible changes to occur before 1 year of age. An understanding of the natural course of pulmonary hypertension is necessary to appreciate its effect on postoperative management. Initially, the elevation in pressure is caused by a marked increase in pulmonary blood flow with essentially normal pulmonary vascular resistance. Eventually, the combination of high flow and pressure through the pulmonary bed leads to pathologic changes in the pulmonary vessels and subsequent elevation of pulmonary vascular resistance. Once this process is initiated, a progressive rise in pulmonary vascular resistance occurs resulting in reduction of pulmonary blood flow. If surgery is performed before the resistance is significantly elevated, the process reverses subsequent to the normalization of pulmonary blood flow and the pulmonary hypertension eventually resolves. However, if surgical intervention is delayed, pulmonary vascular changes progress to a point of irreversibility. Even after successful surgical reduction of pulmonary blood flow, pulmonary vascular resistance and pulmonary artery pressure continue to increase over time. When pulmonary vascular resistance becomes equal to or greater than systemic vascular resistance, right-to-left shunting with systemic hypoxemia results (i.e., Eisenmenger's Syndrome).

In any surgical patient with pulmonary hypertension, problems secondary to hyperreactivity of the pulmonary vessels may occur in the postoperative period. The arteriolar hypertrophy that is universally present allows wide fluctuations in pulmonary vascular resistance and pulmonary artery pressure in response to stimuli such as hypoxemia, hypercarbia, acidosis, and hypoglycemia. Sudden and profound pulmonary vasoconstriction can lead to decreased cardiac output and/or hypoxemia from right-to-left atrial shunting. Treating pulmonary hypertension to avoid these adverse hemodynamic effects includes removal of the predisposing causes. The use of agents to dilate the pulmonary arterioles, such as tolazoline (Priscoline) and sodium nitroprusside (Nipride) may also be useful. As would be expected, the higher the level of pulmonary vascular resistance and the greater the severity of pathologic pulmonary vascular changes that are present preoperatively, the more likely it is that the above problems will occur.

Failure to Thrive and Malnutrition.   These nutritional and developmental consequences of CHF and pulmonary hypertension occur primarily for two reasons. The increased work of breathing in the presence of heart failure leads to increased pulmonary and cardiac metabolic demands. In addition, the intake of nutrients is impaired because of the chronic tachypnea and resultant feeding difficulties. Implications of malnutrition for postoperative management can be profound. Weaning from the ventilator may be impeded because of low energy reserve, wound healing may be impaired, and susceptibility to infection increased. Early aggressive attempts to improve nutrition such as nasogastric tube feedings or hyperalimentation are often necessary to obviate these problems.

Pulmonary Parenchymal Disease.   Pathologic changes in the lung parenchyma can result from cardiac lesions with increased pulmonary blood flow and pulmonary artery hypertension. In fact, the respiratory symptoms along with pulmonary radiographic findings may predominate and mask the underlying cardiac diagnosis. The pathogenesis of these changes includes compression of large airways by dilated proximal pulmonary arteries and enlarged cardiac chambers, compression of small airways by dilated distal pulmonary vessels and peribronchiolar edema, decreased pulmonary compliance from excessive pulmonary blood flow, and increased bronchial secretions secondary to pulmonary vascular congestion.[2,3] These changes result in diffuse hyperinflation, segmental atelectasis or emphysema and a predisposition to pneumonia. The postoperative care of these patients is greatly complicated by preexistant pulmonary disease.

Preoperative Nursing Care.   Prior to surgery the nurse must be alert for signs and symptoms of cardiopulmonary distress. Frequent assessment of respiratory rate is important, since tachypnea is an early indication of CHF or volume overload. Fluid balance can be accurately assessed by measuring weight; such measurements should be obtained daily at approximately the same time with the same scale and amount of clothing. Children with CHF may be more comfortable with the head of the bed elevated or when they are sitting up in an infant seat. Frequent rest periods should be provided with nursing care measures grouped to promote at least 90 min of undisturbed rest. Energy expenditure can be conserved for feedings by avoiding procedures just before or during meals. Oral feeding periods should be limited to 30–40 min, so that caloric expenditure does not exceed caloric value. If the infant has difficulty feeding, both suck and swallow should be evaluated. If the swallowing mechanism seems intact but he has a poor sucking reflex or is easily exhausted, several measures may be taken. Using a softer nipple, a crosscut nipple, or one with an enlarged hole provides faster formula flow. Holding the baby either in an upright position or in a prone knee–chest position may facilitate more intake. Feedings may also be given more frequently in smaller volumes to provide adequate caloric intake. If the infant's condition necessitates tube feedings, a pacifier should be used to facilitate normal sucking. Preliminary studies investigating the use of a pacifier or nonnutritive sucking (NNS) in premature infants suggest that besides facilitation of normal sucking, growth and gastrointestinal function may be enhanced. These findings may have implications for the value of NNS in other groups of high-risk infants.[4,5]

Acyanotic Lesions with Normal Pulmonary Blood Flow

This category mainly includes obstructive lesions on either the right or left side of the circulation. Aortic valvular stenosis (ASV) and pulmonic valvular stenosis (PSV) usually present with a murmur in an asymptomatic child but may be severe enough to cause CHF in infancy. Coarctation of the aorta (COA) may also be severe enough to cause CHF in a young infant, particularly if there is an associated shunt (e.g., VSD, ASD, or PDA). In fact, some of the sickest patients seen in a pediatric cardiology service are 1–3 week-old infants, who have COA and associated VSD. This combination of pressure and volume overload on the left ventricle results in profound CHF, shock, renal failure, and hypoglycemia. Surgical intervention in these patients is urgently needed, but certain preoperative medical measures are indicated for stabilization. These include digitalization, diuretic therapy, reestablishment of glucose and electrolyte homeostasis, and the use of prostaglandins (see Chapter 3). Prostaglandins are remarkably effective in dilating the ductus arteriosus in younger infants, which leads to improved systemic perfusion. Ductal dilatation permits a partial bypass of the obstructing coarctation tissue and thus decreases the extreme afterload on the left ventricle.

Cyanotic Lesions with Decreased Pulmonary Blood Flow

These lesions involve severe right-sided obstruction that results in decreased pulmonary blood flow and intracardiac right-to-left shunting. Tetralogy of Fallot (TOF) is the most common lesion in this category. Patients with TOF that present during the newborn period are usually severely hypoxemic. Metabolic acidosis frequently accompanies the severely depressed PO_2 and should be treated with bicarbonate. Once the diagnosis is established by cardiac catheterization, prostaglandin infusion can be used to increase ductal flow to the lungs and cause a rise of at least 10 torr in systemic arterial PO_2.[6] Such infusions have proved to be tremendously helpful in stabilizing the child prior to surgery. These infants require palliation of their condition by performance of a systemic-artery-to-pulmonary-artery shunt to insure adequate pulmonary blood flow. In the postoperative period, continued use of prostaglandins may help tide the infant through the early period when shunt flow is limited by edema around the anastomosis area. Excessive pulmonary blood flow and CHF are extremely rare with a Blalock-Taussig shunt but can occur with shunts such as the Waterston anastomosis.

Chronic arterial hypoxemia may lead to many complications. Polycythemia occurs as a compensatory mechanism and may become excessive. Marked polycythemia can lead to thromboembolic phenomena and may also be associated with iron deficiency anemia if the child's iron intake is inadequate for the demand incurred by the increased number of cells. The polycythemia can also result in abnormal coagulation. The coagulopathy (prolonged PT and PTT with decreased platelets) may cause hemorrhagic complications in the postoperative period.[7] In addition, because right-to-left intracardiac shunting bypasses the normal filtering system of the lungs, the condition can lead to cerebrovascular accidents or brain abscesses.

Preoperative Nursing Care.   Nurses should observe children with cyanotic heart disease frequently for any of the following symptoms: increasing cyanosis, dyspnea, failure to thrive, diaphoresis, hepatomegaly, squatting, exercise intolerance, and clubbing. Neurologic assessment is crucial because of potential central nervous system complications such as stroke or abscess. Because systemic venous blood bypasses the lungs and goes directly to the arterial circulation, intravenous therapy in these children requires special care. To avoid dislodging small clots or septic emboli, intravenous catheters should not be routinely irrigated. In-line microfilters are preferred and even small air bubbles should be removed from the lines. When children with polycythemia become dehydrated, the risk of thromboembolic complications increases. Therefore, fluid requirements should be accurately maintained and infiltrated IVs restarted quickly. Abnormal coagulation does not usually cause problems prior to surgery. However, nurses should be alert for bleeding and monitor platelet counts. Iron supplements may be necessary if iron intake is inadequate.

Patients with TOF may be susceptible to spasms of the stenosed infundibular area of the right ventricular outflow tract; such spasms result in substantially reduced pulmonary blood flow ("Tet spells"). Putting the child in the knee-chest position increases systemic resistance and may help reverse the massive right-to-left shunting. Additional treatments include administering morphine sulfate to relax the spasm and decrease anxiety and dyspnea, giving bicarbonate to counteract metabolic acidosis, and providing additional inspired oxygen. Propanolol (Inderal) may be indicated for acute dyspneic attacks. Increased frequency of "Tet spells" may necessitate earlier surgical intervention.

Cyanotic Lesions with Normal or Increased Pulmonary Blood Flow

By far the most common lesion in this category is transposition of the great arteries (TGA). A balloon septostomy (Rashkind procedure) is performed in the newborn period and effectively improves arterial oxygenation in most patients for at least several months.[8] When TGA is accompanied by a VSD, severe pulmonary hypertension and heart failure may necessitate palliation in early infancy to reduce pulmonary blood flow (i.e. pulmonary banding). TGA is also commonly associated with pulmonic stenosis in which pulmonary blood flow may be decreased. Infants with this form of defect may require a systemic-to-pulmonary-artery shunt. The majority of patients with transposition undergo an atrial rerouting procedure that utilizes a pericardial baffle (either a Mustard or a Senning operation) some time between 6–12 months of age. The same nursing assessment and care that was described above applies to these patients.

INTRAOPERATIVE TECHNIQUES

Surgical procedures to ameliorate the adverse physiologic affects of congenital heart disease fall into two categories: palliative and corrective. A palliative procedure is one that improves certain hemodynamic parameters and alleviates the resultant symptoms without providing an intracardiac repair. Corrective procedures usually require open heart surgery.

Palliative Operations

A list of the commonly used procedures in this category appears in Table 7-2. The major indications for palliation are an unacceptable mortality associated with repair in infancy and the presence of cardiopulmonary symptoms in a child with an uncorrectable defect.

A systemic-to-pulmonary-artery shunt is frequently required in patients who have severe anatomical obstruction to pulmonary blood flow that is not conducive to repair in infancy (i.e., TOF with severely hypoplastic pulmonary arteries). The most commonly used is the Blalock-Taussig shunt, performed by dividing the subclavian artery and anastomosing the proximal end into the pulmonary artery on the same side. The shunt is preferentially performed on the side opposite the aortic arch.

The other end of the hemodynamic spectrum is when excessive pulmonary blood flow leads to pulmonary hypertension and CHF. If the cause is a large VSD or PDA, the condition may be totally corrected in infancy. However, the mortality for early repairs is prohibitive with lesions such as TGA with a large VSD, some forms of complete ECD, and single ventricle without pulmonic stenosis. In these situations, pulmonary banding is the preferred approach. In

Table 7-2. Palliative Procedures

Indication	Procedure	Specific Technique
Inadequate pulmonary blood flow	Aorticopulmonary shunt	Blalock-Taussig Waterston-Cooley Potts Central
Excessive pulmonary blood flow	Pulmonary banding	
Inadequate interatrial mixing	Enlargement of atrial septal defect	Balloon septostomy Blade septostomy Blalock-Hanlon Open atrial septectomy

this procedure a band of synthetic material is placed around the main pulmonary artery to decrease pulmonary blood flow effectively. If at all possible, total correction is preferable to banding.

Another form of palliation involves enlarging the interatrial defect to allow better crossover of oxygenated blood from the left atrium to the right atrium in infants with transposition of the great arteries. The Blalock-Hanlon operation accomplishes this without the use of cardiopulmonary bypass.[9] Currently, this operation is used very little in uncomplicated transposition in infancy because the results from primary repair are quite good.

Corrective Operations

Closed-heart corrective repairs are possible only with the lesions of COA and PDA. With the exception of in-flow occlusion (temporary occlusion of venous return from the inferior vena cava and superior vena cava allowing a very brief period of time to perform a rapid pulmonary valvulotomy), all open-heart repairs involve the use of cardiopulmonary bypass. The two main approaches are standard bypass and profound hypothermia with circulatory arrest.

Standard Cardiopulmonary Bypass. The purpose of bypass is to make possible a nearly bloodless operative field by artificially taking over heart and lung function and thereby maintaining normal perfusion of the body's vital organs. The basic components of the bypass system include a reservoir to receive all of the systemic venous return, an oxygenator that allows gas exchange and maintenance of physiologic levels of PO_2 and PCO_2, a heat exchanger to regulate temperature of the returning blood, and a pump mechanism to allow perfusion of the systemic arterial system with an adequate pressure.

After median sternotomy and exposure of the heart and great vessels, the venous return is diverted into the heart-lung machine by two separate cannulas placed through the right atrium and directed into the superior and inferior vena cava. Arterial return in young children is directed into the ascending aorta, because the femoral arteries are not of adequate size. The latter are the preferred site for arterial return in adults and larger children. Coronary perfusion is maintained during the procedure except for brief periods of aortic cross clamping. These periods are necessary for critical parts of the repair, since there is considerable venous return from the coronary circulation to the coronary sinus in the right atrium if the aorta is not cross clamped. In recent years, various techniques to improve protection of myocardial tissue during these periods of myocardial ischemia have been developed; they include local hypothermia and use of cardioplegic solutions.[10] If the intracardiac procedure is short, normal body temperature may be maintained. If a longer time is required, mild hypothermia to 28°C (82°F) is used.[11] Full heparinization is required for bypass and is reversed by protamine after bypass is discontinued. At the conclusion of any open-heart procedure, critical air-evacuation maneuvers (i.e., needling of the ascending aorta to prevent air that may have accumulated in the heart from escaping into the arterial circulation) are performed.

Most of the postoperative complications of cardiopulmonary bypass are a consequence of the abnormal physiologic features of circulation via the heart-lung machine. These include (1) low-normal, nonpulsatile cardiac output, (2) local production of metabolic acidosis from areas of poor tissue perfusion, (3) mechanical trauma to blood components, (4) coagulation abnormalities related to platelet destruction and alteration of coagulation factors, and (5) unavoidable embolization of minute amounts of air, fibrin, and particulate material affecting perfusion of the small vascular beds throughout the body. These abnormalities can lead to complications such as hemorrhage from the coagulopathy, acid-base disturbances, and postoperative dysfunction of vital organs such as the lungs, brain, heart, and kidney.[11]

Profound Hypothermia with Circulatory Arrest. Over the last decade extensive experience has been gained in the use of profound hypothermia with circulatory arrest in open-heart repairs.[12-14] This procedure is generally used in children younger than 2 years of age and weighing under 15 kg. It allows removal of all cannulas from the heart and provides a quiet bloodless field for surgical work. The advantages of operating under these conditions when performing an intricate repair of a tiny infant's heart are obvious.

The procedure differs from standard cardiopulmonary bypass in that it requires close monitoring of the core temperature (i.e., use of rectal and esophageal temperature probes), surface and core cooling, circulatory arrest with total exsanguination of the patient's blood into the pump reservoir, removal of the atrial cannula when the repair is performed, and, finally, core rewarming and removal of the patient from bypass. Surface cooling is achieved either by placing the child, wrapped in a protective plastic bag, in an ice pack or by using a hypothermic chamber.[15] The core temperature is lowered to 25°C (77°F) over 30–60 min. At that point, cardiopulmonary bypass is established with the use of a single cannula in the right atrium and a cannula for arterial return in the ascending aorta. The core temperature is then further reduced to 18–20°C (64–68°F; asystole usually occurs around 20°C) and the aorta is cross clamped. At this point perfusion is discontinued, and the patient is exsanguinated through the venous cannula into the pump reservoir.[11-15] Following completion of the repair the patient is transfused with fresh blood prime and bypass is re-established. Gradual core rewarming takes place over 30–45 min and bypass is discontinued at 34°C (93°F). Further warming is accomplished by blankets or heat lamps. The period of time generally considered as safe for circulatory arrest with profound hypothermia is 60 min. If longer periods are required, a brief period of bypass flow can be reinstituted before another period of arrest is undertaken. A technique modification used by some surgeons involves employing moderate hypothermia to approximately 25°C and continuous, low-flow perfusion without circulatory arrest.[16]

The use of profound hypothermia with circulatory arrest is associated with all of the postoperative complications of standard cardiopulmonary bypass plus several others. Glucose homeostasis is considerably disturbed; marked hyperglycemia occurs during the procedure presumably because insulin is inactivated during periods of extreme hypothermia. The hyperglycemia itself rarely causes difficulties but can lead to an exaggerated insulin rebound with a precipitous drop in the blood sugar and profound hypoglycemia in the early postoperative period. Persistent hypocalcemia may also occur. A neurologic syndrome of hyperactivity, choreoathetosis, and seizures may occur several days after surgery. These symptoms are usually self-limited and do not portend permanent brain damage.[11]

Although the concern over possible long-term neurologic sequelae continues, to date extensive follow-up studies have shown no significant incidence of late neurologic complications following profound hypothermia and circulatory arrest.[17] In any child who does not respond appropriately following reversal of anesthesia, a hypoxic central nervous system insult or embolization phenomena should be suspected. The extent of the neurologic deficit cannot be fully assessed until recovery from surgery is complete.

NURSING PRIORITIES IN POSTOPERATIVE MANAGEMENT

Maintaining Pulmonary Ventilation and Gas Exchange

Successful postoperative management of pulmonary function requires control of the airway with an appropriate sized endotracheal tube, close monitoring of arterial blood gases, periodic chest X-rays, and the clinical assessment of breath sounds. Many factors related to surgical intervention can create respiratory insufficiency or depression in the postoperative child. These factors are listed in Table 7-3.

Most patients who have had closed-heart procedures or brief uncomplicated bypass operations will have adequate spontaneous ventilation by the time they reach the ICU. These patients can be removed from the ventilator and successfully extubated within several hours. An oxygen mist environment and frequent pulmonary physiotherapy are important factors in facilitating good pulmonary function.

Table 7-3. Compromising Factors Following Surgical Intervention

Pulmonary Function	Cardiovascular Function
Pre-existing disease	Arrhythmias
Anesthesia	Myocardial ischemia
Microemboli from bypass	Hypovolemia
Pulmonary capillary damage	Tamponade
Phrenic nerve damage	Pulmonary vasoconstriction
Atelectasis	Myocardial pump failure
Hemothorax, hydrothorax	Inadequate repair
Pneumothorax	Malfunctioning prosthetic valve
Pulmonary edema	Metabolic disturbances
Gastric dilatation	Fluid overload
Infection	
Incisional pain	
Fluid overload	

Patients who have had more complex or prolonged procedures require continued ventilation and respiratory mechanical assistance for variable periods of time. This assistance provides an airway in the event of an arrest, facilitates pulmonary toilet, allows the use of sedation, and lessens anesthesia problems if it is necessary to reopen the chest. Both infants who were debilitated and in CHF prior to surgery and those with low cardiac output postoperatively benefit from the decreased work of breathing that is required during mechanical ventilation.

The first priority is always maintenance of a patent airway. If the child is still intubated on arrival in the ICU, the location of the endotracheal tube should be checked immediately. The child should be suctioned within an hour of returning from the operating room and subsequently whenever the secretions are moist. Although suctioning has its obvious benefits, it may lead to hypoxia and vagal stimulation that result in bradycardia or other arrhythmias. Suctioning is safest and most effective when preceded by preoxygenation and physical therapy/postural drainage. If high positive-end-expiratory-pressure (PEEP) ventilation is being utilized, a PEEP device of equal water pressure should be attached to the Ambu bag for preoxygenation. Atelectasis is frequently present following lengthy surgical procedures and may cause fever. Coughing and deep breathing can facilitate better gas exchange and are beneficial for the conscious child who is old enough to cooperate. A pillow held over the incision decreases the pain associated with coughing. Infants and younger children can be sighed with an Ambu bag while they are still intubated. As they recover, they can also be encouraged to exhale through pursed lips. An activity that promotes this is blowing soap bubbles.

Intermittent doses of morphine sulfate should be utilized for sedation for agitation, analgesia for pain, and to prevent the child's bucking the respirator. The alleviation of pain and anxiety may assist in decreasing oxygen needs. However, it should be kept in mind that agitation or anxiety may represent early signs of hypoxia, and therefore, medication should not be administered before cardiopulmonary function is carefully assessed.

Every effort must be extended to keep blood gas parameters at optimal levels. These levels include 7.35–7.45 for pH, 70–100 torr for PO_2, and 30–40 torr for PCO_2. Mild hyperventilation is helpful in decreasing the patient's ventilatory drive when assisted ventilation is used. A chest X-ray should be obtained immediately after the child arrives in the ICU and should be repeated as often as the clinical situation dictates. Chest x-rays are used for the following purposes: to check the position of the endotracheal and other tubes and of the central lines and to detect abnormalities such as atelectasis, pneumothorax, mediastinal hematoma, gastric dilatation, and phrenic nerve paralysis. Bradycardia is an important clinical sign to keep in mind, because its presence is usually associated with hypoxia. The patient should be disconnected from the ventilator and bagged with oxygen while every effort is made to find the cause of the hypoxia (i.e., ruling out mechanical problems such as tube dislodgement or blockage).

Pleural and/or mediastinal chest tubes should be maintained with water seal units and "stripped" or "milked" frequently to prevent clotting. If clots form and obstruct the mediastinal tubes, cardiac tamponade can result. Therefore, the tubes should be stripped, initially perhaps every 5 min and then frequently thereafter. Clots that are noted in the tubing should be immediately removed by stripping. Excessive stripping may result in collapsed tubing because of a build-up of negative pressure. This can be corrected by venting the system. Other safety factors should be noted. Excessive bubbling in the system might indicate an air leak; therefore the system connections should be checked. Conversely, clamping the system should be avoided because tamponade or a tension pneomothorax could result. Finally, after the chest tubes are removed, the child should be observed carefully for changes in respiratory and cardiac status.

A nasogastric tube should be in place to help prevent gastric dilatation while the child is intubated. The tube should be checked for patency at least every 2 hrs and irrigated when necessary. The return of bowel sounds determines when the nasogastric tube can be removed.

Maintaining Normal Cardiac Output

Continual assessment of cardiac output in the early postoperative period is of paramount importance. This is particularly true in patients who were critically ill prior to surgery or in those undergoing prolonged or complex intracardiac repairs. Factors related to surgical interventions that can compromise cardiac output are listed in Table 7-3.

Clinical assessment of physical signs is very important but does not allow the earliest detection of adverse trends. Impaired systemic perfusion results in altered function of the brain, heart, kidney, and skin. Decreased perfusion to the brain is reflected through changes in the level of sensorium. The presence of cardiac ischemia may be indicated by arrhythmias, tachycardia, or bradycardia. Decreased blood flow to the kidneys and skin occurs early with low cardiac output. Urine output should be measured hourly, and oliguria is defined as less than 0.5–1.0 cc/kg/hr. Skin perfusion is assessed by observing color, temperature, and capillary refill. Early vasoconstriction results in cool and pale extremities. As part of the sympathetic compensatory response, the skin may also appear clammy. The findings of cool extremities with poor capillary refill, peripheral cyanosis and mottling, decreased arterial pressure, oliguria, altered sensorium, and thready pulses indicate dangerously decreased cardiac output. Chances for survival are greatly increased if marginal or falling cardiac output is recognized before these physical findings are present.

Early detection of adverse trends in cardiac output can best be accomplished by monitoring multiple physiologic parameters, for which the minimum requirements are an indwelling peripheral arterial line and a central venous pressure (CVP) line. Mean arterial pressure is an important indicator of arterial perfusion, but it must be remembered that this parameter is preserved by compensatory mechanisms until relatively late in the pathophysiologic process of shock. CVP gives some measure of the adequacy of circulating volume and

Table 7-4. Postoperative Monitoring Parameters

Hemodynamic Pressures[a]		Lab Values[a]	
CVP	5–10 torr	Na	135–145 mEq/l
RA	1–7 torr	K	3.5–5.0 mEq/l
RV	15–25 torr	Cl	94–105 mEq/l
PA$_{sys}$	15–25 torr	BUN	6–23 mg%
PA$_{dias}$	8–15 torr	creatinine	0.5–1.5 mg%
		calcium	8–10 mg%
PA(mean)	10–20 torr	glucose	55–200 mg%
LA	6–12 torr	hemoglobin	11–15 gm.
LV	120/10 torr	hematocrit	35–45%
Aorta	120/75 torr	platelets	150,000 cu/mm
MAP	40–70 torr: infants	PT[b]	patient: 11–22 sec
	70–100 torr: children		control: 11–22 sec
CO	2.5 l/min/m²	PTT[b]	patient: 30–50 sec
			control: 30 sec

[a] Values are approximate and may vary with age. Actual *desired* values may also vary with the type of surgical procedure.
[b] Acceptable value ranges.

right-heart filling pressure. CVP and right atrial pressure are essentially equal unless superior vena cava obstruction is present. CVP frequently does not reflect left-sided hemodynamic events. Therefore, when ventricular function is likely to be marginal, measurement of other parameters such as left-ventricular end-diastolic pressure (LVEDP) or left atrial pressure should be added. Significant left ventricular failure can occur without elevation of right atrial pressure. On the other hand, with right ventricular dysfunction, the right atrial pressure may be relatively high in the presence of inadequate left atrial filling pressure. Therefore, either the left atrial pressure or a pulmonary artery line with wedge pressure should be monitored in addition to the CVP or the right atrial pressure. Normal values for the above pressures are listed in Table 7-4. Remember that if the amount of PEEP is greater than 5 cm water, for accuracy, pressure readings should be done with the child removed temporarily from the ventilator.

Direct measurement of cardiac output improves the management of patients with low output states. A thermodilution catheter[18] or the green dye technique[19] can be used for this purpose. The lower limit of acceptable cardiac output is 2.5 l/min/m², and any value below 2.0 l/min/m² is considered critical.[20] If cardiac output is inadequate, blood volume should be expanded (with plasma, albumin, or normal saline if the hematocrit is acceptable and whole blood or packed cells if it is low) until the left atrial pressure is between 15–20 torr and the right atrial pressure 15–25 torr. Once adequate blood volume is achieved, general supportive measures are utilized regardless of the etiology of the low cardiac output. These include use of calcium chloride, catecholamines, and vasodilators (if systemic pressure is not severely depressed). Other possible measures include pacing to optimize heart rate, steroid therapy, and mechanical support such as extracardiac massage or placement of an intra-aortic balloon pump.

A thorough search for the cause of low output is vital, because specific therapy may ameliorate the situation rapidly. Some of the more common causes include inadequate blood volume, cardiac tamponade, arrhythmias and conduction defects, acid–base disturbances, hypoxia, mechanical problems related to inadequate cardiac repair or a malfunctioning prosthetic valve, severe pulmonary vasoconstriction, and myocardial pump failure (related to intraoperative procedures or the presence of profound heart failure prior to surgery). Pump failure may be related to myocardial infarction secondary to coronary artery injury or embolus, ventriculotomy and/or myocardial resection, or prolonged periods of aortic cross clamping with inadequate myocardial preservation techniques. Unfortunately, pump failure because of myocardial dysfunction is one of the most common causes for low cardiac output, and only supportive therapy is available.

It is especially important that the presence of cardiac tamponade (compression of the heart by a collection of blood in the pericardium) be recognized early, since the condition is both life-threatening and reversible. Classic signs indicating the presence of tamponade include markedly distended neck-veins and elevated CVP or atrial pressures in the presence of falling arterial pressure. Pulsus paradoxicus (a greater than 10 torr lowering of systolic pressure during inspiration) and muffled heart tones are also key signs. Other important clues are tachycardia or bradycardia, widened mediastinum on chest x-ray, sudden cessation of chest tube drainage, and precipitous deterioration following removal of monitoring catheters or temporary pacing wires. The treatment consists of rapid transfusion of blood or fluid while immediate preparations are made to reopen the chest and evacuate the compressing hemorrhage or clot. A chest tray should be readily available in the unit, since it may be necessary to open the chest in the ICU before transferring the patient to the operating room. Two units of blood should be available in the unit before intracardiac lines are removed. During the actual removal of the lines, the chest tubes should be stripped vigorously to promote open drainage in the event of hemorrhage.

The child should be assessed for evidence of inadequate repair. CHF may result from a residual shunt or from incomplete relief of obstruction. Persistent or recurrent hypoxemia may also indicate a mechanical problem related to surgery (i.e., a baffle leak in TGA).

CHF usually refers to a more chronic, subacute low-output state that is not of such a degree as to be an immediate threat to life. The causes are often related to myocardial depression from the same factors discussed under the low-output syndrome. The manifestations of systemic congestion include neck-vein distention (or periorbital edema in infants), hepatomegaly, dependent edema, weight gain, and elevation of CVP. Left-sided failure results in pulmonary congestion, râles, tachypnea, frothy secretions, weight gain, and elevated pulmonary artery pressures. The management of this more chronic form of low output includes administering digoxin and diuretics and restricting fluids. Digoxin is more useful here than in the setting of acute critical low-output states where tenuous renal function with electrolyte and acid–base disturbances predispose to digitalis toxicity. The workload of the heart can be decreased through nursing measures such as alleviating pain and anxiety, elevating the head of the bed, and providing periods of rest.

The early recognition of potentially serious arrhythmias is possible through continuous monitoring. Conduction disturbances, tachyarrhythmias, and ectopic beats are common following surgical repairs. Underlying precipitating factors should be searched for and corrected. These include hypoxia, electrolyte or acid-base disturbances (especially hypokalemia and alkalosis), digitalis toxicity, and excessive use of catecholamines.

Third-degree atrio-ventricular block is noted most commonly in surgical repairs that involve closure of a defect in the ventricular septum (i.e. TOF, ECD, VSD) and usually requires at least temporary pacing. Sinus-node dysfunction (especially common following the Mustard procedure) may be manifested by sinus bradycardia and/or prolonged sinus pauses with a junctional escape rhythm. Temporary relief can be obtained with atropine, but pacing may be required.

Supraventricular arrhythmias occur commonly, and the necessity for treatment depends on their hemodynamic consequences. Premature atrial and junctional beats or an accelerated junctional rhythm (with a rate between 100–140 BPM) usually do not require treatment. However, atrial fibrillation or flutter and supraventricular tachycardia commonly result in a rapid ventricular response with adverse hemodynamic effects and do require intervention. Possible treatments include administration of digitalis, edrophonium (Tensilon), or propranolol (Inderal); vagal maneuvers; atrial overdrive pacing; and synchronized cardioversion. Cardioversion is necessary when acute deterioration is present.

Ventricular arrhythmias are potentially more dangerous. Occasional unifocal premature ventricular contractions (PVCs) are usually transient and rarely lead to more serious rhythm problems. However, when PVCs are frequent, multifocal, or occur in salvos (groups of two or more), they may progress to ventricular tachycardia, flutter, or fibrillation. Therefore, they should be treated aggressively. Xylocaine (Lidocaine) is the first-line drug, but procainamide (Pronestyl) or phenytoin sodium (Dilantin) may be required. Rapid ventricular tachyarrhythmias are life-threatening, and immediate cardioversion is indicated.

Pacer wires are sutured in place following complex repairs and should be protected from accidental dislodgment at all times. One method includes placing the wires in a test tube corked with rubber and taped securely to the chest dressing. A rhythm strip should be done on each nursing shift, and a twelve-lead ECG should be obtained each day the child is in the ICU. These strips are analyzed and placed in the child's chart. A temporary pacer with batteries should be available at the bedside during the child's stay. Because battery failure causes a large proportion of pacemaker failure in children, new batteries should be placed in the pacemaker with each child and the pacer labeled with the date and time of battery change.

Cardiac arrest occurs frequently in the critically ill postoperative patient. One of the most common causes for arrest is hypoxia. It may result from mechanical problems with the airway and/or ventilator or from pulmonary abnormalities such as edema, atelectasis, or pneumothorax. Other causes to consider include potassium abnormalities, acidosis, tamponade, or administration of substances such as calcium. The basic approach to cardiopulmonary resuscitation is the same in these patients as in any cardiopulmonary arrest. Internal defibrillation accessories with sterile sternal retractors and chest tray should be available in the unit. If the chest is opened, masks should be worn by all staff around the bed. The ECG and arterial pressure should be observed continuously during the resuscitation effort.

Maintaining of Fluid and Electrolyte Balance

In addition to the obvious potential for development of imbalances in circulating volume following cardiopulmonary bypass and operative blood loss, several physiologic responses of the body to bypass and surgery can complicate postoperative management of fluid and electrolyte balance. A marked tendency to retain sodium and water occurs for the following reasons: aldosterone levels are increased secondary to stress; ADH levels are increased; and fluid is lost into the extracellular fluid space possibly related to altered capillary permeability.[1,20] These factors all explain why restricting sodium and water is very important in the first few days after surgery. It is generally recommended that only 50–75% of maintenance fluid (with little or no sodium) be provided during this period. Infants may be unable to conserve as much sodium and therefore may require some sodium in maintenance fluids.[21]

Accurate weights can provide a fairly reliable assessment of fluid balance. In addition, renal function should be monitored by hourly measurement of urine output, periodic specific gravity and urinalyses, and daily BUN and creatinine levels. A Foley catheter facilitates exact hourly measurement of urine output. All drainage fluids must be accurately assessed. Drainage on dressings and through mediastinal tubes should be weighed and/or measured in ccs. Nasogastric drainage is also an important source of both fluid and electrolyte loss. Blood drawn for routine laboratory studies or blood gas determinations should be included in output totals.

An accurate record of input includes measuring all flush solutions including arterial infusions and solution pushed to clear the line, intravenous maintenance infusions, oral fluids, and administered blood or other colloid products. The fluid used to mix and administer medications should also be counted. If volume is critical, it is possible to use only 1.8cc/hr to flush the arterial line of an infant by employing an infusion pump with the intraflow instead of the pressure bag.

The child's blood balance is determined by comparing drainage via chest tubes and blood samples with the blood products replaced, including packed cells, plasma, platelets, and albumin. Because of the third spacing that occurs during surgery, fluids may reenter the vascular space on the 3rd–5th day postoperatively. During this period the child is especially susceptible to fluid overload if fluids are liberalized too quickly. Therefore, careful fluid assessment should continue throughout the 5th day after surgery.

Blood is sent for laboratory studies immediately following surgery; such studies should include as a minimum assessment of Na, K, Cl, BUN, glucose, and calcium levels, a CBC and differential, a platelet count, and PT and PTT. Laboratory values are checked at least every 4 hrs in the postoperative period, and the staff must be aware of age-related norms (Table 7-4).

Various electrolyte abnormalities are common in the first several days. Dilutional hyponatremia is a common finding and can usually be managed by restricting water, since the total body sodium level is still increased. Hypokalemia is extremely common and results from high urinary excretion secondary to aldosterone effect, administration of diuretics, and the release of cortisol. Every attempt should be made to keep the potassium serum level greater than 3.5 mEq/l. This usually requires high concentrations in the maintenance solution (i.e., 40 mEq KCl/l) in addition to periodic replacement infusions. Electrolyte replacements are given slowly on an infusion pump through deep lines diluted with maintenance solution. Potassium may be safely replaced at a rate of 0.3 mEq/kg/hr. The serum potassium level should be checked and the potassium replaced, if necessary, before the initial postoperative digitalis dose. Hyperkalemia may occur with renal failure following acute low-output syndrome. The rise in serum potassium may be rapid because intracellular potassium is released as the result of cellular damage or acidosis. Hypocalcemia or low ionized calcium may occur, particularly in young infants. It results from the dilutional effects of bypass, large amounts of citrated blood, and the low albumin levels following bypass. Hypocalcemia may lead to seizures or inadequate myocardial function unless it is promptly treated. In the presence of normal protein levels, serum calcium should be kept at approximately 8–10 mg% and may be given in the form of calcium chloride or calcium gluconate at the rate of 20 mg/kg/hr of elemental calcium. Blood levels should be rechecked after calcium replacement.

Glucose homeostasis may be disturbed, especially following profound hypothermia. Infants usually require maintenance solutions containing 10–20% dextrose concentrations, whereas a 5–10% solution is sufficient in older children. Hypoglycemia should be treated promptly with an IV bolus of glucose in a dose of 2–3 cc of 25% dextrose/kg. Any solution with a greater than 12.5% dextrose concentration should be administered through a deep line. Dextrostix are used hourly on infants and on older children until their condition stabilizes. Hyperosmolarity can occur if large amounts of sodium bicarbonate or high concentrations of dextrose are given. Serum osmolarity levels should be checked periodically in such situations.

Appropriate replacement of blood components is an essential part of postoperative fluid management. Clotting studies and blood-volume parameters are monitored closely. For slow blood loss, packed red blood cells are used to maintain a hematocrit of 35–45%. More rapid blood loss requires administration of either whole blood or of packed cells plus replacement of colloid (usually fresh frozen plasma). Hemorrhage may occur from a persistent source of bleeding in the operative field, a coagulopathy, or removal of intracardiac lines. Once coagulopathy is ruled out, reoperation to determine the site of bleeding is indicated if the rate of continued blood loss is greater than 5 cc/kg/hr for 3–4 hrs. If a coagulopathy is present, clotting factor deficiencies and thrombocytopenia should be treated with fresh frozen plasma and platelet transfusions, respectively. A micropore filter made especially for blood products (i.e., Pall filter) should be added to all blood filtration sets because of the massive blood replacement that is required during the operative and postoperative periods.

Maintaining Overall Homeostasis

Additional Metabolic Problems in Infants. Hypoglycemia and hypocalcemia following surgery may be more prevalent in infants than in older children because of immature regulatory mechanisms. Glycogen storage levels are low in stressed cardiac newborns. Furthermore, the additional requirement of heat production following profound hypothermia promotes greater glucose utilization. Another result of hypothermia is the insulin rebound. Because these factors predispose to hypoglycemia, dextrostix should be used every half hour for monitoring until blood levels are stable. Levels lower than 30 mg/100 ml should be treated immediately with a glucose bolus given through a deep line. Hypocalcemia occurs because stores are inadequate, parathyroid function is immature, and endogenous steroid is produced secondary to stress. The symptoms of hypoglycemia and hypocalcemia are similar in infants and include twitching, seizures, and lethargy.

Temperature control is another critical issue for the infant. Heat production in infancy results from an increased metabolic rate that requires enhanced utilization of glucose and oxygen. Cold stress can lead to a metabolic acidosis that causes pulmonary vasoconstriction, intrapulmonary shunting, and increased hypoxia. Thus, inadequate environmental control with resultant cold stress may significantly interfere with maintaining cardiac output and oxygenation. The infant is also predisposed to more rapid water loss through evaporation when overheated because of the large body surface area relative to weight. Obviously, provision of a neutral thermal environment that still allows access for the frequent procedures is desirable. Use of a servocontrolled overhead radiant heat shield provides individualized temperature control, adjustable slanting surface, easy observation, and ready access to the infant. Servotemperature, as well as the infant's skin and rectal temperatures, should be recorded every half hour following profound hypothermia until the child's temperature is stable and whenever vital signs are recorded thereafter. The infant should not be removed from the heat-producing environment until overall homeostasis is achieved.

Physiologic jaundice may occur in a newborn surgical patient and should be treated accordingly. Jaundice may occur in a newborn because of hemolysis of red cells, large quantities of transfused banked blood, and reabsorption of closed-space hemorrhage. Both direct and indirect bilirubin levels should be measured. Nursing care of the infant who has undergone cardiac surgery and then requires phototherapy or exchange transfusion remains the same as for other newborns with jaundice with emphasis on monitoring of blood-volume parameters.

Hyperosmolarity is potentially more dangerous in infants. Rapid changes in serum osmolarity from administration of sodium bicarbonate, high-dextrose concentration, Ringer's lactate, etc., can result in rapid cerebral fluid shifts that sometimes lead to intraventricular hemorrhage. Increases in serum osmolarity greater than 25 mOsm/kg of water in a 4-hr period can be dangerous.[22] If it is necessary to infuse hyperosmolar solutions, they should be diluted and given slowly.

Complications of Specific Repairs. Complications that occur after specific intracardiac procedures are compiled in Table 7-5. The occurrence of complications depends on both the degree of preoperative compromise of cardiac function and the adequacy of the repair.

Psychosocial Implications of Cardiac Surgery. Numerous factors should be considered in assessing the child's reaction to the threat of open-heart surgery. Much research has been done concerning the child's responses during the planned intensive care experience. There is little doubt that the psychologic impact can have a significant effect on physiologic recovery from surgery. The nurse, who spends the greatest amount of time with the child, is the staff member most able to have an impact on psychologic well-being.

The child's developmental level is an important determinant of his psychologic reaction. His perception of the event, his coping mechanisms, and his ability to communicate are also important variables. The ICU experience disrupts some developmental tasks and promotes regression in others. The majority of cardiac surgery patients are very young with limited coping and communication skills. Children should receive age-appropriate teaching in preparation. Assessing the parent's response is paramount, since the young child relies chiefly on the parents for coping. Parent support groups that meet preoperatively help to alleviate some of the natural anxiety, answer questions,

Table 7-5. Frequent Complications of Specific Repairs

Defect	Complications
ASD	Air embolism
	Atrial arrhythmias
VSD	Heart blocks
	Residual shunts
TGA (Mustard or Senning Procedures)	Supraventricular arrhythmias
	Sick sinus syndrome
	Superior vena cava obstruction
	Pulmonary venous obstruction
	Tricuspid regurgitation
TOF	Residual pulmonic stenosis
	Congestive heart failure
	Heart blocks
	Inter-atrial shunting
COA	Paradoxic hypertension
	Spinal cord damage
	Mesenteric arteritis
	Chylothorax
TAPVR	Persistent pulmonary edema
	Low output syndrome
ECD	Mitral insufficiency
	Heart blocks

and prepare the parents psychologically for the upcoming surgery. A tour of the ICU before surgery is an effective way for the primary nurse and parents to become acquainted and share information. The child may be involved in the "tour" by way of photographs or filmstrips. Social work support is very helpful, especially when the child is subjected to repeated hospitalizations. Other factors to assess include the child's past responses, the special fears and fantasies of the child, and the child's understanding of the problem.

Some of the disruptive influences in the ICU cannot be completely eliminated by the nurses. These include sensory overload (technical equipment, lights, noise, etc.), sleep deprivation, fast-paced movements, intermittent separation from family, care by multiple strangers, pain, frequent invasive procedures, change in sensorium, and powerlessness of the child to control his environment. These factors caused Berlin[23] to describe an "ICU syndrome" in children aged 18 months–6 years. This syndrome is characterized by severe passivity, withdrawal, and decreased responsiveness to the environment. Behavioral changes, nightmares, and even hallucinations have been reported following ICU care. For this reason, continued professional support after discharge may be helpful in reducing parental anxiety.

Nursing interventions may alleviate some of the stress inherent in pediatric ICUs. These interventious are as follows:

1. Assigning primary or continuity nurses
2. Ensuring that age-appropriate preoperative preparation is given to the child and the parents
3. Providing security for the child by allowing frequent parent visiting/ support, permitting security objects in bed, and accepting coping mechanisms
4. Facilitating communication especially while the child is intubated through techniques such as use of a "magic slate" and picture cards, consistent use of names, and announcing one's presence at the bed
5. Providing appropriate "normal" stimuli and decreasing noxious stimuli by use of familiar objects and family tape recordings, reality orientation, frequent explanations, shielding the child from traumatic events in the unit, avoiding bedside medical discussions and limiting repeated physical exams by students
6. Providing periods of rest and sleep at least 90 min in length[24] by clustering nursing procedures, dimming lights at night, organizing the daily routine, administering pain medication, and awakening the child before painful procedures are done
7. Involving the family in care as much as possible by supporting parents, allowing them to verbalize, showing the child pictures and tapes of siblings, and allowing the family to hold the child when possible
8   Providing opportunities for appropriate play and activities when the child is ready

Although tremendous progress has been made in improving survival of critically ill children after cardiac surgery, many physiologic and psychologic crises remain inherent to the perioperative period. Since approximately 90% of the direct postoperative observation and care of these patients is performed by the nursing staff in the ICU, the nursing role in perioperative management is both critical and challenging.

REFERENCES

1. Sade RM, Cosgrove DM, Castaneda AR: Heart surgery for infants. In: Infant and Child Care in Heart Surgery. eds. Sade RM, Cosgrove DM, and Castaneda AR. Chicago, Year Book Med Pub, 1977 pp 15–23
2. Hardof AJ, Mellins RB, Gersony WM, Steeg CN: Reversibility of chronic obstructive lung disease in infants following repair of ventricular septal defect. J. Pediatr 90:187, 1977
3. Oh KS, Park SC, Galvis AG, et al.: Pulmonary hyperinflation in ventricular septal defect. J Thorac Cardiovasc Surg 76:706, 1978
4. Bernbaum J, Pereira GR, Watkins JB: Nonnutritive sucking (NNS) enhances maturation of the sucking reflex in premature infants. Pediatr Res 15:477, 1981
5. Bernbaum J, Pereira GR, Watkins JB, Peckham GJ: Enhanced growth and gastrointestinal function in premature infants given nonnutritive sucking (NNS). Pediatr Res 15:650, 1981
6. Lewis AB, Takatiashi M, Luri PR: Administration of prostaglandin E_1 in neonates with critical congenital cardiac defects. J. Pediatr 93:481, 1978
7. Wedemeyer AL, Edsen JR, Krivit W: Coagulation in cyanotic congenital heart disease. Am J Dis Child 124:656, 1972
8. Neches WH, Mullins CE, McNamara DG: The infant with transposition of the great arteries II. Results of balloon atrial septostomy. Am Heart J 89:603, 1972
9. Ochsner JL, Cooley CA, Harris LC, McNamara DG: Treatment of complete transposition of the great vessels with the Blalock-Hanlon operation. Circulation 24:51, 1961
10. Kirklin JW, Conti VR, Bluestone EH: Prevention of myocardial damage during cardiac operations. N Engl J Med 301:135, 1979
11. Sade, RM, Cosgrove DM, Castaneda AR: Cardiopulmonary bypass and hypothermic arrest in infants. In: Infant and Child Care in Heart Surgery. eds. Sade RM, Cosgrove DM, and Castaneda AR. Chicago, Year Book Med Pub, 1977 pp 41–52
12. Castaneda AR, Lambert J, Sade RM, et al.: Open heart surgery during the first three months of life. J Thorac Cardiovasc Surg 68:719, 1974
13. Sade RM, Williams RG, Castaneda AR: Corrective surgery for congenital cardiovascular defects in early infancy. Am Heart J 90:656, 1975
14. Subramanian S: Cardiac surgery in infancy using deep hypothermia. In: Current Problems in Congenital Heart Disease. eds. Eldredge WJ, Goldberg H, and Lemole GM. New York, SP Med Scient Books, 1979 pp 35–46
15. Subramaniam S: Hypothermia and Circulatory arrest In: Pediatric Surgery. eds. Ravitch MM, Welch KJ, Benson CD, et al. Chicago, Yearbook Med Pub, 1979 pp 593–597
16. Smith DL, Wilson JM, Ebert PA: Cardiac surgery in infants up to one year old. Cardiovasc Med, 1978 vol 3, pp 925–944
17. Subramanian S: Sequellae of profound hypothermia and circulatory arrest in infants and small children. In: The Child with Congenital Heart Disease after Surgery. eds. Kidd BL and Rowe RD. New York, Futura Pub, 1976 p 421

18. Freed MD, Keane JF: Cardiac output measured by thermodilution in infants and children. J Pediatr 92:39, 1978
19. Bradley EC, Barr JW: Fore-'n-aft triangle formula for rapid estimation of area. Dye dilution curve. Am Heart J 78:643, 1969
20. Aberdeen E: The care of infants and children after heart operations. In: Pediatric Surgery. eds. Ravitch MM, Welch KJ, Benson CD, et al. Chicago, Yearbook Med Pub, 1979 pp 598–611
21. Behrendt DM, Austin WG: Management of infants. In: Patient Care in Cardiac Surgery. eds. Behrendt DM and Austin WG. Boston, Little Brown, 1980 pp 57–78
22. Finberg L: Dangers to infants caused by changes in osmolal concentration. Pediatrics 40:1031, 1967
23. Berlin CM: The pediatric intensive care unit. Med Ann DC, 39:486, 1970
24. Sanford SJ: Sleep in the critical care setting. In: Current Practice in Critical Care. vol. 1, St Louis, CV Mosby, 1979

8 Cultural Considerations in the Care of a Critically Ill Vietnamese Child and Family

Marie Moore
Christine Garvey

Nancy Stanish
Elaine Dobbins

Ma, ma! Däu! Däu! Däu! Con Dė Nha. Om em. What do these phrases mean to you? Translated, they probably mean, "Mommy, mommy! It hurts! It hurts! My head hurts. I want to go home. Hold me. Mommy, it hurts!" These phrases might be what a small frightened Vietnamese child would say when sick and in pain.

Try to imagine yourself a child—sick, hospitalized, and alien to the strange unpredictable environment where no one speaks or understands your language or knows your culture, beliefs, and traditions.

One patient population that we are beginning to see more frequently in our critical care units is that from southeast Asia. This group is comprised of different nationalities—Vietnamese, Cambodians, and Laotians. Unknowingly, people often lump these cultures together. Although the overall culture we are seeing is Asian, both differences and similarities exist between the subgroups. This chapter will specifically address refugees from Vietnam, many of whom the media have dubbed the "boat people." These refugees have immigrated from a once independent and developed (but now war-ravaged) country to the United States with high expectations and heavy responsibilities. They are faced with the challenge to retain their identity and cultural beliefs while adapting to the ways of another people.

The Indochinese refugees have brought with them potential health problems—diseases that have been fairly well controlled or eradicated in the United States. According to the Center for Disease Control, tuberculosis (TB) is the most serious potential health problem in this group. Almost 50% of adult refugees from southeast Asia have positive skin tests.[1] One reason for the positive tests is that western practitioners have given most adults bacille Calmette-Guerin (BCG) vaccine in an attempt to provide artificial immunity for tuberculosis. Another reason for the increased incidence is the crowded living conditions, first during the war in refugee camps in Vietnam and then in resettlement apartments in the United States. One-third of those adults with positive tests have been treated for active TB. Approximately 1% of this group will develop TB meningitis. Unfortunately, the Center for Disease Control does not have statistics on the incidence of TB in the children of Indochinese refugees. However, the crowded living conditions have increased the risk of exposure to TB in these children. Although any age group can develop the disease, teenagers are the most susceptible (see Community Health, Education and Resources).

The purpose of this chapter is threefold: to review the concept of transcultural nursing through an exploration of the cultural beliefs of the Vietnamese people; to discuss the acquisition and transmission of the tubercle bacillus organism; and—as an example of critical care nursing with children of a culture different from that of the provider—to review pediatric TB meningitis in the context of pathophysiology, chemotherapy, and cultural considerations for nursing care.

"Transcultural Nursing" is a term coined by Dr. Madeline Leininger in her book *Transcultural Nursing Concepts, Theories and Practices* and is defined as "the area of nursing which focuses upon the comparative study and analysis of different cultures and subcultures with respect to nursing and health care practices, beliefs, and values with the goal of generating scientific and luministic knowledge and of using this knowledge to provide cultural specific and cultural universal nursing care practices."[2] Dr. Leininger has identified the need for nursing education that focuses on people of the world with respect to their cultural beliefs including health care values.[3] Unequivocably, knowledge of one's own culture is necessary for holistic patient care. Without awareness of cultural differences, the patient may be misunderstood and may not be cared for sensitively or totally. Through greater sensitivity to and awareness of such differences, cultural conflict can be decreased and nursing care can be given more effectively.

THE VIETNAMESE CULTURE

The Vietnamese people have experienced several governments over the last 130 years. It is particularly important to note that Vietnam has been the center of international controversy since World War II and has had to fight the longest and hardest of all the countries (over 100) that have won independence from colonial rule. At the risk that a sketchy and oversimplified view will be presented, only the primary powers will be highlighted. However, the bibliography provides excellent sources for a more in-depth study of Vietnam's intense and complicated political and economic history.

In the mid-nineteenth century, France annexed "Vietnam" and renamed it French Indochina. During French colonization, Vietnam was one of the most stable, developed, and sophisticated of the southeast Asian countries. Western colonization was basically directed at the maintenance and function of a capitalist economy. The development of the Vietnamese Communist Party in 1930 laid the foundation of protest against French rule and colonialism. In 1954, France finally withdrew after a shattering military defeat at Dien Bien Phu, the capitol of "North" Vietnam, and Vietnam became an independent country, although divided into northern and southern regions. The United States, which had become a major Pacific power after World War II, moved in and filled the vacuum created by the French withdrawal from Indochina. US military involvement deepened in southeast Asia, and Soviet and Chinese support prevailed in North Vietnam. The cease-fire agreement was signed in January, 1973 and the United States eventually withdrew. In 1975, the Vietnam People's army overtook Saigon, and a provisional government was established. This event abruptly ended two centuries of western involvement in southeast Asia, but the vicious power struggles between capitalism and communism continued.

As the country was ravaged by war, the rural farmers and peasants fled from their farms and rice paddys to the cities, one of which was Saigon, the capitol of South Vietnam. However, one group of people was driven in the opposite direction. In Vietnam, the merchants were often Chinese and were commonly referred to as the "Jews of the Orient." Because they were hated for political and economic reasons, they were forced through the countryside to the sea. There, the Chinese merchants could afford passage to escape and became what we know as the "boat people."

Since 1975, numerous Indochinese refugees have sought haven in twenty-eight countries, including the United States and its territories. California, with 69,652 refugees, has absorbed the majority of those choosing to come to this country from Indochina. But a brief survey of other states shows that the influx has been both widespread and considerable: Texas (20,949), Pennsylvania (9,562), Louisiana (8,309), Washington (8,009), Illinois (7,340), Virginia (7,264), New York (5,856), Oregon (5,680), Minnesota (5,508), Florida (5,475), and Colorado (4,734).* The magnitude of these figures has many implications for

---

* The Newest Americans. Newsweek, 25, 1979.

the importance and necessity of cultural awareness in nursing, especially when we realize that they apply to only one of the many groups of people seeking refuge here.

The next section reviews aspects of the Vietnamese culture to allow for more sensitive consideration and care while their children are hospitalized.

Philosophy of Religion

Historically, spirituality has been a powerful force for southeast Asians. Buddhism specifically has been a factor in the life of the nation currently known as Vietnam. Buddhism provides a value for individual responsibility and states that life is repeated on and on. Thus, how one lives a current life will affect his next life. Although French influence brought about the conversion of many Vietnamese to Roman Catholicism, Buddhism remains the predominant religion today. Of course, secularism has increased with the exposure of many Vietnamese to city life and western culture.

General Buddhist guidelines for living include beliefs such as:

Moderation and the middle path is best.

Self-denial and overindulgence are both negative.

Reincarnation is a basic fact of life.

Life is a succession of suffering caused by desire for happiness, riches, and power.

Confucianism has also had a strong influence over the Vietnamese. Its main ethics are Jen, which represents benevolence or humility, and Shu, representing tolerance or reciprocity. Confucius strongly believed that social and family order could be attained by involvement with music, adherence to social rites, and respect for authority.[5]

Taoism, another strong influence, is characterized by a belief in numerous gods. Its philosophy focuses on the relationship between man and the universal order—that is, achievement of harmony between man and man and between man and nature. This order is exemplified through an equilibrium between Yin (negative) and Yang (positive) elements. Man seeks contentment in nature, quietness, and a peaceful mind.[4]

A small percentage of the Vietnamese people are Roman Catholic; however, they have played an important role in both the cultural and the political life of Vietnam.

In addition to the above-mentioned sources of influence, the Vietnamese people also believe in good and evil spirits, or animism. The belief in astrology, fortunetelling, omens, and natural signs may be strong. Therefore, when problems arise, a diviner may be consulted to determine which spirit is angry and which ceremony might appease him.[6]

Family

The basic unit in the Vietnamese society is the extended family, which includes more than one generation: grandparents, married sons, daughters-in-law, grandchildren, and aunts and uncles. All members may live within one household and respect towards elders is expected. The senior male acts as head of the household and the Vietnamese male must be consulted in any dealings with his family. Many Vietnamese consider sons more desirable than daughters because they carry on the family line and work to support the family.

In contrast, women are concerned with household chores and childcare. Mothers care closely for their children during the first 2 years of life, after which grandmothers and aunts assume greater responsibility for their care. Children are not over-indulged and are encouraged to begin caring for themselves at an early age. As with any country in war, women have assumed more responsibilities out of the home as men have left to fight. Thus the family structure seen in young families is very different and one may see real "generation gaps."

Social Status

Within the Family.   Traditionally, the Vietnamese have been concerned more with status than with wealth. Social and family heirarchies exist to maintain order, and the family heirarchy is based on one's relationship to other family members in terms of sex, age, generation, paternal or maternal side, and marriage. The Vietnamese husband heads the family, earns the income, makes the decisions, and has a higher status than his wife. He gives her money to pay for food and other expenses, and she gives him pocket money in return. Parents commonly support their married children financially. With respect to assets, it has been inconceivable for the husband and wife to have separate bank accounts and properties.

Vietnamese women have a low status in society. Women are taught three basic principles while still under their parent's protection: they must obey their fathers, be submissive to their husbands after marriage, and listen to their grown-up sons when they become widowed. Consequently, the role of women is predominantly confined to childbearing and rearing. However, with the increase in widowhood after war, role changes may be seen.

Vietnamese children are subject to strict discipline. They must obey and respect all older people, even their oldest siblings. Children are expected to help with babysitting, cooking, cleaning, and other household chores. When the parents become too old to work, children proudly take care of their parents.

Within Society.   As in many other societies, Vietnam has social class divisions based on differences in religious, political, educational, social, and economic status. The society consists of a small educated elite, a nominal middle class, and a large uneducated peasantry. The refugees from rural regions are primarily rice farmers and fishermen with little education. The difference between urban and rural background may be more significant than a particular national background.

Education

Many criticisms have been levied on the Vietnamese system of education for its lack of diversity and availability to the general population, and for the resultant high rate of illiteracy. Despite these concerns Vietnamese people highly value education, because it determines an individual's self-esteem, social status, and the honor that is bestowed on his family.

In general, Vietnamese education is based on three principles: humanism, nationalism, and open-mindedness. The humanistic aspect aims at full sacred development of man; the nationalistic viewpoint emphasizes respect for traditional values; and the open-mindedness component permits acceptance of all cultural values of the world.

Primary education is mandatory for all children ages 5–10 (5th grade). There are both public and private schools, and government-supported universities have been established in recent years. The basic subjects are language (Vietnamese), moral education, civics, history, geography, mathematics, science, home economics, and child care.

The educational process used in Vietnamese schools emphasizes rote-learning instead of problem-solving. Students are taught to observe rather than to discover or experiment. Emphasis is placed on memorization and repetition rather than on open discussion and study. The teacher's authority is acknowledged by students and parents alike. Questioning the teacher's knowledge or the presented material is unacceptable, and parents do not become involved in school activities.

Hygienic Habits

The Vietnamese environment is tropical, providing high temperatures with frequent heavy rainfall. People wear light cotton clothes and rubber shoes. Houses vary from modern apartments to open-air bamboo and wood huts. Toilet facilities also vary widely from modern enclosed tiled bathrooms in the cities, through rain barrel showers and "squat" toilets (which may be porcelain), and finally to primitive body cleansing and elimination in open areas. The likelihood of diseases such as hepatitis, malaria, intestinal parasitic disorders, and tuberculosis is great.[7]

Several hygienic habits of the Vietnamese stem from their traditional beliefs, which are often rooted in myths and folklore. Among these is the belief that women should not bathe or shampoo their hair following delivery of a baby. They believe that too much water to the body causes the woman to lose nutrients and energy through her skin and probably leads to illness.[8] The emphasis on myths and the lack of facilities potentiates the transmission of contagious disease.

Dietary Preferences

Because the Vietnamese are generally small in physical stature, fewer calories are required daily. Foods are simple. The diet is based on a staple of rice, meat (mainly pork or chicken) or fish, vegetables, and other preferred foods such as soups with noodles, coagulated blood from animals, fruits, and green tea.[9]

Particular foods are omitted or included from the Vietnamese diet for specific reasons. Dairy products are eaten by only a few because most Vietnamese suffer from a lactase deficiency that prevents the digestion of milk.[10] Salads are believed to cause diarrhea, and beef and seafood are believed to promote itching. Diarrhea might occur because fresh vegetables are not adequately washed or cooked. Foods that are eaten for specific reasons include bitter melon to refresh the stomach and intestines and red peppers (eaten frequently) to prevent worms. The Vietnamese promote health by drinking alcoholic preparations from porcupine belly or snake and by eating salty foods and pork to restore health.

The temperature of food is important to Vietnamese people. They believe that food must be hot to keep the stomach warm and to counteract heat loss. They also believe that cold foods and cold water are bad for the teeth and stomach.

Their diet is based on moderation and balance, in accordance with their philosophy of life. A proper diet includes balanced portions of "hot" (Yin) and "cold" (Yang) foods. "Hot" foods include fish sauce, spices, onions, and peppers, whereas "cold" foods include rice, noodles, meats, fish, and potatoes. When Yin and Yang foods are not in balance, a person is considered susceptible to disease. The Vietnamese traditionally eat twice a day and the main part of the meal is a bowl of rice with a portion of anything that is left over from the meal before. A favorite sweet consists of rice cooked in syrup and wrapped on a stick.

American life may influence Vietnamese body structure and diet. Although Vietnamese are small in stature, the size may at least partially reflect an unavailability of food. Studies may indicate growth in stature with changes to western eating habits. Most Vietnamese children in America ravish sweet foods, especially candy and soda. Besides, they are influenced by peer pressure to eat what the other kids eat.

Language

Several languages are spoken in Vietnam. Although Vietnamese predominates, English and French may be spoken by the elite or the educated. In addition, Chinese is a common language in business.

Although the origin of the Vietnamese language is unclear, it has borrowed from the Chinese language. It has used the Chinese system of writing (using characters) and has borrowed and changed the pronunciation of words. Vietnamese is a tone language—that is, each symbol has a musical pitch or tone that determines interpretation of the word. Recently, the Chinese writing system has been modified to incorporate selected letters from the Roman alphabet. Another language characteristic is that names are written in a different order from that used in the West, for example, Vuong Gia Thuy (family/middle/given) is in contrast with John Joseph Smith (given/middle/family).

Perspectives in Health

The Vietnamese concepts of health and illness are influenced by their religious and cultural beliefs. In the Buddhist belief, sickness may result because an individual or family member was bad in this or his previous life. Ill health may therefore be considered preventable or a punishment. Vietnamese also believe the holistic concept that health depends on a balance of negative (Yin) and positive (Yang) forces within the body, and that this balance maintains immunity and prevents disease. Improper diet and strong emotions are two factors that may disturb this balance. Other cultural beliefs include concepts about touching. One shoulder of a person must not be touched without touching the other; to touch only one shoulder disturbs the spirits and bestows bad luck. Touching a person's head (especially that of adults and older children) should be avoided because the head is linked with one's ancestors. That is, the head is symbolic of the sacred ancestral spirits, and touching violates or angers the spirits.

When a Vietnamese person becomes ill, he believes that he is responsible for curing himself. Therefore, he only seeks professional help when home remedies fail. These remedies may include herbs, potions, broths, meditation, or spirit-removal ceremonies. Sorcery is used to frighten away the evil spirits believed to cause mental illness. Remedies such as antibiotics from Indochinese pharmacies are used to supplement home remedies. Traditionally, the family cares for its ailing member[11] and avoids hospitals when possible. If hospitalization is necessary, a family member must remain close and cook for the patient.

Death and Dying

Like all people, the Vietnamese are grief-stricken in the face of death. The loss of a family member is particularly devastating. When hospitalized and dying, patients usually prefer to leave the alien environment of the hospital and die at home. In addition, the relatives consider that they violated their culture to take the patient to the hospital, and they prefer to remove him and to practice their rites and rituals within the familiar surroundings of their own home.

These perspectives of Vietnamese culture establish a framework for interacting with and caring for the Vietnamese child and family. Application of many of these concepts will be further discussed in the section on nursing considerations.

TUBERCULOSIS MENINGITIS

Pathophysiology

The term tuberculosis refers to all the tissue changes caused by Mycobacterium (myco is from the Greek *mykes,* meaning fungus or mold) tuberculosis—the tubercle bacillus; the bacilli causing tuberculosis and leprosy are two pathogenic species among numerous nonpathogenic species of Mycobacterium. Tubercle bacilli can be inhaled or ingested and can colonize in almost any tissue and organ system. The most common variant is pulmonary TB, and thus the lungs are considered the primary site.

TB is called a granulomatous disease because normal tissue respond to invasion of the organism by forming new tissue masses that are called infectious granulomas. Two tissue reactions can occur in response to the tubercle bacillus. In the first, a localized response, a tiny spherical infectious granuloma, called a tubercle or little tumor, is formed. In the second, more diffuse reaction, the bacilli travel with the lymph and blood streams and lodge in small clumps in susceptible tissues. Neighboring tissues may successfully form a protective wall to arrest the spread of the bacteria and kill them over a long period of time via an effective immune system. If this defense process succeeds, the tubercle transforms into a tiny mass of fibrous tissue. Otherwise, the tissue of the tubercle necroses and caseates (transforms into a cheesy mass). Necrosis and caseation liberate the bacilli, and they are swept into surrounding tissues that respond by enclosing them in new tubercles.

TB meningitis is caused by the transportation of the tubercle bacilli from the lymph system to the spinal canal. The tubercle bacilli lodge in the meninges where caseation occurs, the tubercle bursts, and tubercle bacilli enter the subarachnoid space. Infection develops, adhesions form, and neurologic complications appear.[12] These are caused by edema, adhesions, or infarction of the brain.

Diagnosis

The importance of early diagnosis of TB meningitis cannot be overemphasized in relation to initiation of treatment and prognosis. Making the diagnosis may be difficult because symptoms may be misleading in the early stages. The prodromal phase of TB meningitis usually occurs 2–3 weeks prior to the appearance of overt symptoms. The child may have personality changes, malaise, apathy, low-grade fever, and an isolated seizure. The signs are often missed because they are intermittent. The prodromal phase may also pass unnoticed. Following the prodromal phase, the child presents with fever, headache, and intermittent vomiting. He may complain of an earache, abdominal pain on the lower right side, or joint pain. Diseases such as otitis, appendicitis, and rheumatism must be ruled out. Neurologic symptoms such as photophobia, neck stiffness, and change in level of consciousness generally do not appear until the later stages of the disease.

Unless treatment is begun in the early stages, the disease may progress to the point where the child exhibits personality changes and becomes hostile, irritable, and drowsy. Diagnostic signs consist of localized seizures, hemiplegia, and ocular paralysis. Brain-stem involvement may be exhibited by both abnormal respiratory patterns and by changes in the pulse rate and cardiac rhythm. Lethargy generally progresses until coma supervenes. The child may become non-responsive and have a fixed stare and dilated pupils. Seizures may continue with the appearance of opisthotonos and decerebrate posturing. Finally, death may occur by asphyxiation.

This reiterates the importance of early diagnosis and treatment. Patients with TB meningitis have a focus of primary tuberculosis elsewhere (usually the lungs) and present with the disease 6–12 months after infection.[13]

Treatment

The treatment for TB meningitis must be started immediately. Tuberculosis is rarely treated by a single antitubercular drug, because resistant strains of

Table 8-1. Drugs Used in the

Drug	Adult Dose	Child's Dose	Selected Characteristics
Isoniazid (INH)	5 mg/kg/day up to 300 mg, PO, NG or IM in single or divided doses Miliary or meningeal TB: initially 7 mg/kg/day for 7–10 days, then 3–5 mg/kg/day	10–30 mg/kg/day up to 300–500 mg PO, NG or IM in single or divided doses	Primary antitubercular agent Most effective tuberculostatic agent Effective against rapidly growing tubercle bacilli Higher doses recommended in children and young adults because drug is inactivated faster in these groups Well-absorbed from the GI tract and it's injection site Well-distributed through most tissues
Rifampin (RIF)	600 mg/day PO in a single dose	>5 years of age 10–20 mg/kg/day, not to exceed 600 mg/day PO in a single dose	Primary antitubercular agent; semisynthetic antibiotic Bacteriostatic and bactericidal activity that interferes with metabolism of bacteria Well-absorbed from GI tract Well-distributed throughout all body tissues and fluids
Streptomycin	1 g/day IM in single or divided doses	30 mg/kg/day IM in single or divided doses	Antibiotic, aminoglycoside antibacterial Rapidly distributed throughout most tissues and body fluids including necrotic tubercular lesions

the disease exist. Concomitant use of two or three drugs guards against this problem. Currently, the favored triad of primary agents is isoniazid (INH), rifampin (RIF), and streptomycin. Substitution of one or more of these drugs with secondary agents such as ethambutol or ethionamide is determined by the child's degree of improvement and CSF and sputum-culture results. Ethambutol has recently replaced para-aminosalicylic acid (PAS) as the drug of choice for noncavitous disease. See Table 8-1 for further antitubercular drug infor-

Treatment of TB Meningitis

Contraindications	Side Effects	Nursing Implications
Severe hypersensitivity to isoniazid To be used with extreme caution in patients with seizure disorders Lowest dose possible in patients with impaired renal function	Excess CNS stimulation; seizures may occur at higher dosage levels Peripheral neuritis; parasthesia, optic neuritis and atrophy Toxic psychosis Hyper-reflexia Ataxia Drowsiness, excitement, euphoria Delay in micturation Dry mouth Hematologic and hepatic changes	Observe malnourished clients more carefully because neurotoxic reactions are more marked in them. Have parenteral sodium phenobarbital available to control INH-induced neurotoxic symptoms, especially seizures. Monitor periodic ophthalmoscopic exams and hematologic and liver function results.
Hypersensitivity to rifampin To be used with extreme caution in patients with hepatic dysfunction	GI upset: heartburn, epigastric distress, anorexia, nausea, vomiting, flatulence, cramps, and diarrhea Headaches, drowsiness, dizziness, mental confusion, visual disturbances Fatigue, ataxia, muscle weakness Pruritis, urticaria, purpura, and skin rashes Low-frequency hearing loss Hematologic changes and liver dysfunction Casts in urine	Check for GI disturbance, impaired renal function, auditory nerve and visual impairment, and blood dyscrasias. Inform client and family that rifampin colors urine, feces, saliva, sputum, and tears orange. Observe for jaundice due to liver dysfunction. The drug may interfere with hepatic uptake of bilirubin and result in excessive unconjugated bilirubin, causing jaundice. Thus, the jaundice is due to liver dysfunction, not liver necrosis.
Hypersensitivity to streptomycin Contact dermatitis Exfoliative dermatitis Existing myasthenia gravis or renal insufficiency	Ototoxicity (8th CN), disturbance of vestibular function Damage to optic nerve; conjunctivitis Blood dyscrasias Pain and tenderness at injection site Renal irritation Peripheral neuritis, neuromuscular blockade, and apnea with parenteral administration are reversed by neostigmine	Observe for side effects and discontinue streptomycin if headache, ataxia, or other vestibular signs such as high-pitched tinnitus (ringing in ears) appear. The latter foreshadows auditory damage. Protect clients with vestibular dysfunction: supervise ambulation and provide side rails. Monitor I&O because decreases in renal function may result in a cumulative effect. Tell the client and family that auditory dysfunction is cumulative and may manifest for up to 6 months after the drug has been discontinued

Table 8-1.

Drug	Adult Dose	Child's Dose	Selected Characteristics
Ethambutol	15 mg/kg/day for 10–12 days PO in a single dose	>13 years of age: same as adult <13 years: contraindicated	Primary antitubercular agent, tuberculostatic Arrests multiplication of tubercle bacilli Does not affect tubercle bacilli during their resting state Has replaced PAS as the drug of choice for noncavitous disease
Ethionamide	0.5–1.0 g/day PO in single or divided doses	>12 years of age: 12–15 mg/kg/day up to 750 mg PO in single or divided doses <12 years: contraindicated	Secondary antitubercular, antituberculostatic agent Readily absorbed after PO administration Potentiates CNS toxicity of cycloserine
Cycloserine	250 mg/12 hr PO for 2 weeks, if tolerated, increase to 250 mg/8 hr 250 mg every 6 hr sometimes required to maintain blood levels of the drug at 20–30 μg/ml	Not recommended in children because of insufficient data	Secondary antitubercular agent Believed to interfere with the formation of the bacterial wall Readily absorbed from the GI tract

mation and implications for nursing. Other drugs that are sometimes used are anticonvulsants, barbiturates, diuretics, and steroids for neurologic involvement; antipyretics for hyperthermia; and antiemetics for gastrointestinal disturbances. In addition to definitive and adjunctive chemotherapy for TB meningitis, supportive therapy includes replacing body fluids and maintaining nutrition, aiding respiration, minimizing seizure activity, and relieving brain-tissue swelling.

Although the antitubercular drugs available to treat TB meningitis are effective, late diagnosis and treatment and resistance to the drugs may affect the prognosis. If treatment is initiated prior to the onset of neurologic symptoms, improvement—evidenced by relief of headache, vomiting, and drowsiness—may be seen within 1 week. The fever, however, may persist up to 4 weeks. In contrast, if treatment is started after neurologic symptoms appear, improvement may be slow and may depend on the amount of damage caused

(continued)

Contraindications	Side Effects	Nursing Implications
Hypersensitivity to ethambutol To be used with caution and reduced dosages in patients with gout, impaired renal function, and pregnancy	Ocular toxicity: optic neuritis, decreased visual acuity, loss of color (green) discrimination, temporary loss of vision or blurred vision Renal damage, hyperuricemia Anaphylactic shock Decreased liver function Peripheral neuritis (rare)	Test patient for visual acuity and check for pre-existing visual problems before starting ethambutol. The patient should have a vision test every 2–4 weeks while on therapy. Reassure the patient and family that the eye effects usually resolve within several weeks to several months after therapy has been discontinued. Observe I&O in patients with known renal damage for systemic accumulation of the drug.
Children <12 years of age unless primary treatment has failed	Gastric irritation: anorexia, nausea, vomiting, upper abdominal discomfort, and diarrhea Neurologic effects: metallic taste, sialorrhea (salivation), mental depression, drowsiness, asthenia (weakness), severe postural hypotension, headache, and peripheral neuropathy Acne and skin rash Jaundice and hepatotoxicity	Observe for toxic effects, especially severe nausea, which can be treated with antiemetics. Check urine of diabetic clients more frequently and observe for side effects related to diabetes. TB makes diabetes more difficult to control. Observe for potentiation of toxic effects of cycloserine (CHF) if that drug is given concommitantly.
Hypersensitivity to cycloserine Epilepsy, depression, severe anxiety, psychosis, severe renal insufficiency, alcoholism	CNS neurotoxicity: drowsiness, dizziness, headache, mental confusion, tremor, lethargy, allergic dermatitis, photosensitivity, psychotic reactions, anxiety, seizures (petit and grand mal), liver damage, and peripheral neuropathy. Neurotoxic effects depend on blood levels of cycloserine. (see Adult Dose)	Monitor blood levels of cycloserine frequently, especially during the initial period of therapy. Observe for sudden development of CHF in clients receiving high doses of cycloserine. Observe for side effects, especially the neurologic ones that will require withdrawing the drug for at least a short period.

Adapted from Loebl S, Spratto G, Wit A, and Heckheimer E: The Nurse's Drug Handbook. New York, John Wiley and Sons, 1980, pp 99–100; pp. 131–140

by the adhesions or edema. Regardless of the course, antitubercular drug therapy must continue for 12–18 months to cure TB meningitis.[14]

NURSING CONSIDERATIONS IN CARING FOR THE CRITICALLY ILL VIETNAMESE CHILD AND FAMILY

Application of Cultural Considerations

Although patients with TB meningitis may be admitted to the hospital during any point of the disease, the Vietnamese child is often admitted in the late phase. This delay occurs because of cultural beliefs about illness and home remedies and because the parents may not understand the disease course or the need for hospitalization. They may not notice the often intermittent signs of the prodromal phase or may try to treat the symptoms with home remedies that may include employing a sorcerer to remove the evil spirits thought to cause a seizure or personality change. They may also believe that the child's ill health is caused by either his or a relative's bad behavior in this or a previous life or that the balance of Yin and Yang forces within the body are upset. Also, the family will only seek professional help when everything else is attempted and fails. Unfortunately, this delay often results in a critically ill child who requires physical isolation, noninvasive and invasive monitoring, and, frequently, mechanical ventilation. Regardless of the delay in seeking hospitalization, the family should be treated with respect. They may be asking for help after they have exhausted all of their familiar cultural efforts to cure the child.

Admission of a Vietnamese child to the ICU can be an extremely unfamiliar and traumatic experience for the child, family, and staff. However, certain measures may lessen the impact of this experience and make it more positive. When the unit is informed of the pending admission, those in charge should try to learn the child's age, religion, who is with him, and who his sponsoring agency is, in addition to other pertinent information. Every refugee must have a sponsor or agency who provides support services and assigns interpreters and social workers. The support services include job training and teaching English.

Interpreters are essential in caring for the Vietnamese family. Interpreters can be obtained through the sponsoring agency or through a 24-hr hotline that some states, such as Pennsylvania, have established. These names and telephone numbers should be included in the kardex and posted at the child's bedside. Learning to work with an interpreter is complex and a skill in itself. Some beginning pointers are (1) to face the client while speaking through the interpreter, (2) to speak slowly and clearly, and (3) to use visual aids if appropriate. It is also important to realize that the translations may appear different from your stated directions. Inaccurate translations may occur because of insufficient knowledge of English, misunderstandings, and personal interpretations including omissions and embellishments, among other reasons. Therefore, it is important to develop a good working relationship with the interpreter, that is, one built on trust over time.

If possible, arrange for an interpreter to be present on the child's arrival and throughout the admission events. Communication about the child's status (such as asking questions and providing information while taking the history, during orientation and teaching sessions and when updating the family) should be directed to the father. Questions about the family's former life style and adaptation to American life are very appropriate. The child's mother may also be approached, but she will probably feel uncomfortable being "confronted" (answering questions or receiving information) in the absence of the father. However, if it is necessary, she may feel more comfortable speaking with a female interpreter because of the Vietnamese concerns for status. It is also important to know that the Vietnamese may avoid eye contact in a situation of authority—a consequence of the Asian value of humility. They may be shy or embarrassed, because only peers are entitled to make direct eye contact. Knowledge of the family's religion (which may not be recorded on the admission form) may provide a basis to understand their beliefs, actions, and expectations, and to develop a nursing-care plan.

Other actions may help break through the communication barriers. Primary care givers should learn the words that are most frequently used and attempt to speak Vietnamese. Such an attempt will be greatly appreciated despite a limited vocabulary or a poor accent or inflection. These efforts may demonstrate sincerity and help to foster trust—the most difficult value to earn. Words can be learned in both languages by using aids such as a Vietnamese–English dictionary and a chart with corresponding words and pictures. The guide compiled by Smith-Santopietro and Dobbins[16] provides a basic vocabulary of general and health-related terms. A chart with body pictures is helpful with procedures, bodily functions, and ailments. Nonverbal communication including gestures, facial expressions, and touch should be used as much as possible to convey emotions and activities.

The Vietnamese child and family, as with any family, need understanding, support, orientation, and education throughout their hospital experience. However, because experiences of the hospital and western culture sharply contrast with their eastern culture and beliefs, special concern and attention is necessary. Consistent medical and nursing (especially primary nursing) care for the Vietnamese child and family may help to generate familiarity (with personnel, customs, and the hospital), trust, *reciprocity*, and cooperation, and may decrease fears and confusion. Trust is the most important element and may never be achieved because of the cultural differences.

Awareness and respect for nuances of Vietnamese culture may help generate trust. Several diverse considerations follow. Vietnamese react to the stress of illness in character with their heritage. If they believe that the child's illness is caused by an imbalance of Yin and Yang (bad and good), they should be permitted to continue their familiar cultural practices such as administering potions and summoning a diviner. Because some Vietnamese believe that life is a succession of suffering, they may appear to accept illness more readily than others. This may be evidenced by family members who do not express emotion. However, support and guidance should be continued despite this appearance. Other nuances reflect status and interaction. Since the Vietnamese father is the decision-maker of all family affairs, doctors should discuss the child with him. Because the Vietnamese are taught to observe and not question (the teacher's knowledge), they also assume that health care professionals are authoritative and they therefore may not volunteer information. Thus, the health-care team should be very direct and ask the child and family questions. Furthermore, information should be repeated frequently. This repetition is important because of the language and culture barrier, the effects of anxiety and stress on the ability to concentrate and comprehend, and because Vietnamese education emphasizes repetition, memorization, and role learning. A caution that is basic to many cultures is never to mistake a smile for understanding. It is also important to be careful about where and how the Vietnamese—especially adults and older children—are touched with respect to their head and shoulders.

Health-care personnel should be particularly aware of some of the commonly used folk medicine practices and resultant misconceptions by westerners. Some Asians have been suspected of child abuse[17,18] because multiple bruises are seen on their children in the emergency room. The bruises, however, are a form of folk medicine. If the family practices folk medicine, a person in the neighborhood may be assigned to that role. The bruises are created by pinching the skin in symmetrical designs and by coining—in which a hot coin is dipped in salve and the skin is scratched until it turns red over the chest, neck, arms, and back in a symmetrical design (almost like a bib). These practices are similar to catharsis, or burning the bad out of the person. The salve may also be applied to different parts of the body, and the coin may be worn on a string around the neck. Another folk medicine therapy is used to try to draw out head pain. A lighted match is briefly put to the forehead while a small glass or cup is put over it to create a vacuum and leave a mark. Other practices are innocuous. Amulets (coins, metals, keys) are worn to "lock out death," and multiple strings are tied in knots around the wrist as a symbol of confining the protective spirits inside the body and warding off the evil spirits. It is important to realize that it is an insult to cut off the strings. If their removal is necessary, ask the child's mother for permission. A comfort measure akin to the western custom of patting the head is rubbing the skin—especially that of the extremities. Touch is very important to the Vietnamese. Additional cultural considerations are interspersed throughout the remaining discussions.

TB Testing and Isolation Considerations

When taking the child's history, one should also obtain a complete family history to determine the mechanism of transmission of the initial infection and to provide information for public health follow-up. All family members should be tested for the disease. They should first be taught about required procedures for themselves and their child and the necessity for them. Once Vietnamese understand what is required, they will most likely consent because they believe they are responsible for their own fate.

Testing for tuberculosis can be done with the Mantoux Tuberculin Skin Test, which involves inoculation of tubercle bacillus extract into the inner aspect of the forearm. Either Purified Protein Derivative (PPD) or Old Tuberculin (OT) is injected intradermally, and the site is checked 48–72 hrs later for signs of an inflammatory response that is evidenced by the extent of induration or hardening. A positive TB test, represented by an inflamed area 5 mm or greater in diameter, indicates that a person has either had contact with the tubercle bacillus or has been vaccinated with BCG. A positive response signifies little about the activity of the infection. Generally, however, a more intense reaction denotes a greater likelihood that the disease is active. A person suspected of having an active infection may have an intense reaction to the testing. Therefore, it is customary to start the testing by injecting very dilute or "first strength" PPD and successively increasing the dose if negative reactions occur. A negative test has greater diagnostic value, because it almost rules out the presence of active TB except in specific circumstances.[15]

Other diagnostic measures include chest X-rays, sputum smears, and a lumbar puncture. The latter, whereby the cerebral spinal fluid (CSF) is tested for tubercle bacillus, is the diagnostic tool for TB meningitis.

When TB meningitis is suspected, isolation precautions should be taken until the diagnosis is either ruled-out or confirmed and the organism is no longer evident in the cultures. The child should be placed in appropriate room isolation to prevent the spread of the bacterium to other patients, staff, family, and visitors. Because TB is communicated through respiratory droplet, blood, stool, and urine, isolation measures should include donning of isolation gowns, gloves, and masks by all people in contact with the isolated child and by strict observance of handwashing before and after each contact with the child.

The alien environment of the hospital becomes even more bizarre when isolation procedures are instituted. Depending on his condition the child may be overwhelmed by feelings of loneliness caused by separation from his extended family. Furthermore, the gowns, gloves and masks are at once intrusive and a barrier to interaction and may compound the separation anxiety. The family should be taught why the measures are necessary and how to carry them out. This information may be established by the physician through the interpreter and elaborated on by the nurses, also through the interpreter. The family will most likely learn the techniques well because they learn by observing, role modeling, and repeating. Even though they may not understand, believe, or accept concepts about western medical practices (e.g., germ theory of disease), they will respect the authority of the profession, especially because their traditional practices have failed. The family will explain what they feel is appropriate to the child—again, depending on his condition. This explanation should be known by the staff. If possible, there should be a list of interpreters who are available for each shift. In many cities the Office of Refugee Resettlement provides interpreters who are available by phone and who are also willing to come to the hospital. A patient care conference should be held with the primary nurse, all auxiliary services, the family, and the interpreter within the week of admission and perhaps weekly or more often depending on the circumstances and the child's condition.

Isolation is stressful for anyone, but isolation in a strange place with unfamiliar people and medical practices and frightening equipment is traumatic. Furthermore, separating a critically ill Vietnamese child from his family disrupts many of their ways of life. Although the child's grandmother usually stays with the child 24 hours a day, each member of the large, extended family may provide support for the ill and isolated child and should be encouraged to be involved in his care, if appropriate. Visiting hours should be flexible to accommodate and support the needs of the child and family.

Nursing Interventions

Nursing interventions for the Vietnamese child with TB meningitis must be based both on a thorough knowledge of the disease entity and its potential pathologic effects and on an understanding of the child's cultural background. The nurse must integrate the child's available history and unique cultural characteristics with clinical findings and laboratory data and must act to prevent system failure and promote health. The following discussion highlights nursing interventions and certain cultural considerations specific to those interventions. More thorough discussions of assessments, interventions, and physiology can be found elsewhere.

An essential nursing intervention to determine the child's status and prevent undesirable sequelae is to do a baseline assessment and then continual follow-up studies of systems and age-appropriate behavior (Table 8-2 shows age-appropriate vital sign values). Detailed flowsheets are necessary to determine trends and to provide prompt and early intervention.

Neurologic assessments determine the extent of alterations in the neurologic status caused by increased intracranial pressure (ICP). Criteria include level of consciousness (arousability, lethargy), pupil size and reaction, reflexes, spontaneous movements, extremity strength, head circumference, and fontanelle contour. Continual assessment of the head is more difficult if ICP monitoring is necessary because of the Vietnamese belief that the head (especially in children over 7 years old—the age of reasoning) should not be touched. Careful communication is essential in explaining the need to break this taboo and in supporting the family to earn their trust. Another area of difficulty is the occurrence of seizures. Vietnamese believe that seizures are caused by evil spirits and therefore may summon a diviner to rid the spirits or may put a special object in the room to stop the seizure and cure the disease. Allow this, but at the same time, negotiate a compromise to conduct assessments and other interventions in conjunction with their familiar practices.

Assessments to evaluate the effect of increased ICP on the respiratory system include observation of rate and rhythm, skin color, chest excursion and symmetry, nasal flaring and the use of accessory muscles, and auscultation for the quality and characteristics of breath sounds. Intubation and mechanical ventilation may be necessary and may upset the family even more because of the equipment and the necessity for more frequent touching of the head to carry out routine tracheal toilet and, if indicated, hyperventilation for increased ICP.

Circulatory system assessments determine the extent of alterations in circulatory status caused by effects of increased ICP on the brain stem, and possible thrombus, anemia, and hypovolemia. These assessments include evaluating heart rate and rhythm, color, peripheral pulses (presence, quality, and equality), and blood pressure—especially for widened pulse pressure. Evaluating intake and output is also important.

Subacute sepsis commonly occurs with TB meningitis. Therefore, frequent temperature monitoring is necessary. Hyperthermia warrants a complete septic

Table 8-2. Normal Vital Sign Ranges in Children*

Temperature**

Oral	36.4–37.4°C (97.6–99.3°F)
Rectal	36.2–37.8°C (97–100°F)
Axillary	35.9–36.7°C (96.6–98°F)

Age	Normal Respirations/Min
Newborn	30–50
6 months	20–30
2 years	20–30
Adolescent	12–20

Heart Rate at Various Ages

Age	Heart Rate/Min Mean	Range
Term Newborn***		
0–24 hours	145	80–200
1–7 days	138	100–188
8–30 days	162	125–188
1–3 months	161	115–215
3–6 months	149	100–215
6–12 months	147	100–188
1–3 years	130	80–188
3–5 years	105	68–150
5–8 years	105	68–150
8–12 years	88	51–125
12–16 years	83	38–125

(Adapted from Ziegler RF: Electrocardiographic Studies in Normal Infants and Children. Springfield, Charles C Thomas, 1951; from a table appearing originally in Homans J: Textbook of Surgery, 6th ed., 1948. Courtesy of Charles C. Thomas, Publisher, Springfield, Ill.)

*** Editor's note: Many clinicians request that early bradycardia (pulse under 100) be reported in infants up to 1 year old.

Normal Blood Pressure for Various Ages

Age	Mean Systolic ± 2 S.D.	Mean Diastolic ± 2 S.D.
Newborn	80 ± 16	46 ± 16
6 months–1 year	89 ± 29	60 ± 10
1 year	96 ± 30	66 ± 25
2 years	99 ± 25	64 ± 25
3 years	100 ± 25	67 ± 23
4 years	99 ± 20	65 ± 20
5–6 years	94 ± 14	55 ± 9
6–7 years	100 ± 15	56 ± 8
8–9 years	105 ± 16	57 ± 9
9–10 years	107 ± 16	57 ± 9
10–11 years	111 ± 17	58 ± 10
11–12 years	113 ± 18	59 ± 10
12–13 years	115 ± 19	59 ± 10
13–14 years	118 ± 19	60 ± 10

(Adapted from Haggerty RJ, Moroney MW, Nadas JS, et al.: Essential hypertension in infancy and childhood. AMA Journal of Diseases of Children, 92:536, 1956. Copyright 1956 American Medical Association.)

Head and Chest Circumference

Age Yr. Mo.	Head Circumference Inch	Cm.	Chest Circumference Inch	Cm.
Birth	13.8	35.0	13.0	33.0
3	15.9	40.4	15.8	40.2
6	17.1	43.4	17.1	43.4
9	17.8	45.3	18.0	45.7
1–0	18.3	46.6	18.6	47.3
1–6	18.9	47.9	19.4	49.2
2–0	19.3	48.9	19.8	50.4
3–0	19.6	49.8	20.6	52.5
3–6	—	—	20.8	52.8
4–0	19.8	50.4	21.0	53.4
5–0	20.0	50.8	21.5	54.6

(Data From Studies at Harvard School of Public Health)

* Adapted from: Brunner LS and Suddarth DS: Pediatric Physical Examination. In: The Lippincott Manual of Nursing Practice 3rd edn, Philadelphia, JB Lippincott, 1982, pp 1067–1068
**Adapted from: Brunner LS and Suddarth DS: Pediatric Physical Examination. In: The Lippincott Manual of Nursing Practice, Philadelphia, JB Lippincott, 1974, p 1067

workup (cultures of blood, urine, stool, and CSF) and administration of anti-pyretics. Hypothermia may be used for temperatures above 39.4°C (103°F).

Provision of adequate nutrition and fluids is hampered by the increased demands made by the illness, the severity of the child's condition, and the availability of culture-specific food. The services of an interdisciplinary nutrition support team may be necessary if the child is NPO for three (3) days or more. A dietician should be involved in the child's care either to provide or to supplement the cultural requisites of food variety, taste, and dietary balance of Yin and Yang foods that are believed to maintain and restore health. Of course, the family may bring in home-cooked food. The child's inability to ingest food and his need for nutritional support through parenteral and enteral routes may be more upsetting to the Vietnamese than to us because of their beliefs regarding the association of foods with health and illness.

As mentioned earlier, the prognosis depends on when the treatment was initiated and on its effectiveness. If permanent neurologic impairment occurs, physical and occupational therapy may be required for rehabilitation. If death is imminent, the parents and family should be allowed to stay with the child and practice any of their cultural beliefs.

Community Health, Education, and Resources

Follow-up care is essential to prevent a relapse of the disease process, to educate the child and family, and to identify potential sources of transmission. The best way to achieve successful follow-up is to make an early and positive connection with the sponsor. It may also be accomplished with the help of interpreters through visits to the clinic or visits from community health nurses. The most important fact the family must learn is that the antitubercular medications must be taken for 12–18 months after their initiation to cure TB meningitis. Home visits may be necessary to foster compliance, especially when there is a tendency to stop taking the drugs when the child feels better.

The family also needs to be taught about the disease process—preventive measures, the importance of recognizing the symptoms and seeking medical help early (in spite of their cultural beliefs), and of follow-up examinations for the child, family members, and contacts. This is especially important because of the high incidence of positive skin tests and treatment for active TB among Indochinese refugees. Furthermore, exposure to the disease is compounded by the close contact associated with their extended family structure. So, it is likely that an entire family(ies) need ongoing and long-term follow-up.

Because artificial immunity has been attempted without success,[19] the only way known to prevent TB is to avoid contact with infected persons. However, resistance can be built against the tubercle bacillus by getting adequate nutrition and sleep, by avoiding debilitating infections, and by avoiding drinking milk that is not pasteurized. The latter point may be less of a concern; unpasteurized milk is not that easily available and few Vietnamese drink milk, because they are lactase deficient.

Tuberculosis can develop in any age group. Children exposed to individuals with active TB should be examined yearly. Vigilance should be especially increased during adolescence, because the child is most susceptible to the disease then.[15] Moreover, adolescence is when old infections are likely to reactivate and new ones are likely to occur.[15] This has special implications for teaching and screening.

Although health care and education may be a challenge because of language and cultural differences, certain characteristics of the Vietnamese people portend a successful outcome. Their ability to learn well and their belief that ill health can be prevented and that they are responsible for their own destiny are strong indicators for learning and compliance within our unfamiliar culture.

Community outreach programs and refugee-help groups may be instrumental in education, prevention, and assistance with medical bills. Other support sources may include the Regional Director of the Office of Refugee Resettlement, the Department of Health and Human Services, state and local health departments, and the Tuberculosis Association. Health education of the Vietnamese family and public is inherent in its prevention and reoccurrence. All health care professionals involved with the Vietnamese should be sensitive to their culture, and be creative and flexible in meeting their needs. It is also important to note that the incidence of tuberculosis in the Indochinese refugee is not as high as feared.

CONCLUSION

Perhaps no other group of recent refugees has endured such profound suffering and culture shock as the Vietnamese boat people. Health professionals have many responsibilities for these refugees. One of the biggest tasks is to become familiar with their culture, beliefs, and traditions. Another major task is to realize that many cultures exist in Vietnam; that many similarities exist among these as well as other Asian cultures; and that the similarities and differences should be considered in the care of these groups. By studying the multiple aspects of the Vietnamese people, we can intervene to provide comprehensive health care. It is necessary for the nurse of the 1980s to understand the disease process, to perform physical assessments, and to participate in interventions, rehabilitation and health teaching where major cultural barriers exist.

REFERENCES

1. Center for Disease Control, Morbidity and Mortality Weekly Report 28:385, 1979
2. Leininger M: Transcultural Nursing Concepts, Theories and Practices. New York, JW Leg and Sons, 1978
3. Leininger M: Transcultural nursing for tomorrow's nurses. Imprint 25:44, 1978
4. Stringfellow L, Nguyen DL, Diepliem L: The Vietnamese in America. In: Culture and Childbearing. ed. Clark AL. Philadelphia, FH Davis, 1981
5. Vuong GT: Getting to Know the Vietnamese and Their Culture. New York, Frederick Ungar Pub, 1976

6. Dobbins E, Lynch BA, Fischer DK, Smith-Santopietro MC: A beginner's guide to Vietnamese culture. RN, 44(1):45, 1981
7. Koval D, Brennan AMW: Exotic diseases you're sure to see more of. RN, 43(9):73, 1980
8. Hollingsworth A, Brown LP, Brooten D: The refugees and childbearing. RN, 43(11):47, 1980
9. Crawford A: Customs and Cultures of Vietnam. Mt. Pelier, Vt, CE Tuttle, 1968
10. Dobbins E, Lynch BA, Fischer DK: Translating the Indochinese diet into English. RN, 43(9):79, 1980
11. Shubin S: Nursing patients from different cultures. Nursing 80:79, 1980
12. Brunner LS, Emerson CP, Ferguson LK, Suddarth DS: Patients with pulmonary tuberculosis. In: Textbook of Medical Surgical Nursing. ed. Intenzo D. 2nd edn. Philadelphia, JP Lippincott, 1970, p 298
13. Parsons M: Tuberculosis Meningitis, A Handbook for Clinicians. Oxford, Oxford Press, 1979
14. Gerbeaux J: Types presenting with meningeal TB. In: Primary Tuberculosis in Childhood. ed. Kugelmass IN. Springfield, Ill., Bannerstone House, 1970, p 298
15. Brunner LS, Suddarth DS: Infectious Diseases. In: The Lippincott Manual of Nursing Practice. ed. Intenzo D. Philadelphia, JB Lippincott, 1974, p 1022
16. Smith-Santopietro MC: How to get through to a refugee patient. RN, 44(1):47, 1981
17. Gellis SS, Feingold M: Pseudobattering in Vietnamese Children. Am J Dis Child 130:857, 1976
18. Yeatman GW, Shaw C, Barlow MJ, Bartlett G: Pseudobattering in Vietnamese Children. Pediatrics 58(4): 616–618, 1976 (has a photograph of symmetrical purpura caused by coin rubbing)
19. Marlow DR: Long-term conditions of the adolescent patient. In: Textbook of Pediatric Nursing, 4th ed. Philadelphia, WB Saunders, 1973, p 717

SUGGESTED READINGS

Benda HJ and Bastin J: A History of Modern Southeast Asia: Colonialism, Nationalism and Decolonization. Englewood Cliffs, Prentice-Hall, 1968

Butlinger J: Vietnam: The Unforgettable Tragedy. New York, Horizon Press, 1977

Committee of Concerned Asian Scholars: The Indochina Story. New York, Bantom Books, 1970

Dawson A: 55 Days: The Fall of South Vietnam. Englewood Cliffs, NJ, Prentice-1 808Hall, 1977

Hall, 1977

*Garrett WE: Asia's homeless: Thailand, refuge from terror. National Geographic, 157:633, 1980

*Grant B: The Boat People: An "Age" Investigation. New York, Penguin Books, 1979

*Hanh TN: Vietnam: Lotus in a Sea of Fire. New York, Hill and Wang, 1967

Maclear M: The 10,000 Day War: Vietnam. New York, St Martin's Press, 1981

Marshall SLA: West to Cambodia. New York, Cowles, 1968

*Rosenblatt R: Children of War. Time, 119:32, 1982

*Thomas L: Dust of Life. New York, Dutton, 1978 (A Nurse's Mission to the Children of Vietnam)

---

* Recommended

9 | Care of the Critically Ill Child—Is There a Better Way?

Janet L. Snow

The care of critically ill children has over the last several years become an art unto itself, advancing by leaps and bounds. Although pediatrics has been established as a specialty for over 50 years, subspecialization within pediatrics is a new concept. Critical care pediatrics is only now emerging as a viable subspecialty for both physicians and nurses. It is interesting that the benefactors of recent therapeutic breakthroughs and accompanying technological advances have been of two different age groups, namely, adults and newborn infants. Today there are approximately 1400 adult intensive care units (ICUs) in the country and 200 neonatal intensive care units (NICUs) employing approximately 2800 and 500 medical intensive care specialists respectively, not to mention thousands of nurses.[1]

Care of the critically ill child has not been acknowledged as a priority, and thus care has remained relatively unorganized and essentially unimportant in the eyes of the medical and nursing world. Even the technologists have expressed little enthusiasm about developing pediatric-oriented equipment, thereby making it impossible at times to acquire equipment specially designed for children.

The focus of this chapter will be to highlight what exists today in terms of care of the critically ill child and what needs to be done to ensure (from this author's viewpoint) quality care of critically ill children in the future.

The concept of a critical care unit that has been developed specially for children (PCCU) was conceived in the early to middle 1960s. Small units of two to four beds were created adjacent to pediatric units primarily to care for children who needed more than routine nursing observation. Children with respiratory disorders such as croup or with contagious diseases were segregated into a room with one nurse. The rooms also served as glorified postanesthesia recovery rooms. The units were not sophisticated in design and often lacked even the basic monitoring equipment so common to critical care today. As more and more children underwent surgery for congenital heart defects, these units often became postoperative step-down areas for the children after they left the adult ICU.

Pediatric ICUs began to flourish in the early 1970s. Today it is estimated that there are approximately 115 pediatric ICUs; one associated with each medical school in the United States.[1] The units vary in size and service. Some units consist of as few as two beds, others as many as 30 beds; some provide care for children with multiple trauma or needing postoperative cardiac care, whereas others are equipped to care for children with tracheostomies and central intravenous lines.

In spite of the ever increasing number and size of pediatric ICUs, progress towards caring for critically ill children is disappointing compared with the progress registered in the last 5 years in neonatal and adult critical care.

MANPOWER NEEDS IN PEDIATRIC CRITICAL CARE

Manpower needs exist at both the medical and nursing level. A conservative estimate is that two medical intensivists are needed to administer each unit. In light of the approximately 115 pediatric ICUs nationwide,[1] approximately 230 positions are potentially available for pediatric-trained intensivists. Currently, approximately 50 physicians are known to be practicing pediatric intensive care medicine nationwide. Furthermore, at the present time only 12 training programs exist for physicians in pediatric critical care in America compared with approximately 27 training programs for adult intensivists.[1]

The numbers in nursing are even more dismal. Although there are graduate programs in nursing geared to training adult and neonatal specialists, not one (1980) has provisions for advanced didactic and clinical practice in pediatric critical care nursing. The average pediatric ICU consists of six beds. (Snow J, unpublished survey, 1970). The ideal minimum number of nursing personnel necessary to staff the average unit is 18 nurses, which allows for 1:1 nursing care around the clock. Nationwide then, the ideal minimum number is somewhere in the range of 3000–3500 nurses.

As the number of infants surviving life-threatening disorders continues to increase, it is most probable that the number of children requiring critical care will increase. Disorders such as respiratory distress syndrome and necrotizing enterocolitis have created a whole new population of children with bronchopulmonary dysplasia and nutritional problems, many of which require intensive and step-down care for some time after their initial hospitalization. As a result, many of the pediatric ICUs are expanding from their original pre-1970 bed complement to accommodate the increasing numbers of critically ill children. As this occurs, the need for skilled nurses and step-down units will certainly increase.

Furthermore, the demographic trends show a changing age mix in the United States. Between now and the year 2000, the number of children from 1–12 years of age is expected to increase by at least 13%. However, the age group between 13–24 years is expected to decline (by approximately 1.5%).[2] The elderly population, on the other hand, will increase in number approximately 35% from the present level. The baby boom of the 1940s will leave a population predominately in the 35–64-year age range.[2] The future birthrate is unpredictable, but some speculators believe another baby boom is imminent. A higher birthrate may indicate a need for expanding the current number of pediatric critical care beds.

ALTERNATIVES FOR CARING FOR CRITICALLY ILL CHILDREN

Children are not all cared for in pediatric ICUs. The adult ICU is accepted as standard in almost any hospital today; and in many general hospitals, children are cared for alongside of critically ill adult patients.

Children certainly can and do survive in a setting outside of the pediatric department. In fact, the idea of one ICU to accommodate all critically ill patients (except neonates) is not a new one. Many children, even today, spend their first few days after major surgery in the adult surgical ICU. Does it really make a difference where a critically ill child is cared for? The idea of an alternate approach to the pediatric ICU can be more fully explored by looking at the issue from different viewpoints.

Quality of Care

Caring for children is a unique and challenging experience (see Chapter 10). The care is complex in that most pediatric ICUs are general units, accommodating all sorts of cases from trauma to medical crises, and surgical insult to burns, rather than any one entity as is the case in some adult ICUs.

In addition to the complexity of caring for the critically ill child, the nurse must deal with the wide age range. The pediatric ICU may encompass children from the newborn period up through young adults of 25 years of age. Growth and development issues are a major consideration in the care of children. A neonate, for example, requires different handling from that needed by a 3-year-old. The same is true for a 6-, an 8-, or a 12-year-old. There is no standard piece of equipment for pediatric patients. Most equipment is useful for children of a particular age or size. For example, diapers come in at least five sizes, suction catheters in at least six, and endotracheal tubes in at least eight. Vital sign parameters are also dependent on growth and development. A pulse of 140 may be quite normal for a newborn but would indicate marked tachycardia in a 6-year-old. A blood-pressure reading of 60/40 may be fine for a newborn but indicates gross hypotension in a 10-year-old child.

The dosage and administration of medications are still other examples of the complexity within pediatrics. A particular drug dosage may be very appropriate for one child of a certain age but grossly inappropriate for another child who is the same age but who weighs less. Intravenous fluid maintenance is yet another example. A 2-kg child may have a daily fluid requirement of only 200 ml, whereas a 5-kg child would need 500 ml. A small amount more or less could make a significant difference. Nothing can be taken for granted in the pediatric ICU. Virtually every treatment, drug, and piece of equipment requires a nursing judgement prior to its use.

Psychologically, the separation of a child from his family during a crisis is an important issue to consider (see Chapter 7). A child depends on his parents as the main resource for coping in all stages of development, and the reaction of the child to the absence of his parents may greatly affect his physical well-being. Parental visiting privileges in pediatrics have been liberalized in recent years, with most hospitals across the nation permitting 24-hour visiting.[3] However, in some ICUs the length of stay is limited. Because of the parents' importance to the child, great lengths are taken to make the parents comfortable in the ICU. In many cases, the parents are involved in the care and become valuable members of the team.

Nurses do not experience the same kind of growth and developmental problems with adults as are experienced with children. Without a background in growth and development, coupled with in-depth pediatric nursing knowledge, nurses who are oriented to the care of adults become focused on dealing with the physiologic consequences of the disease process.

A good example would be the case of a 2-year-old boy who has had open heart surgery. The child returns from the operating room with an endotracheal tube and two mediastinal chest tubes in place. The child is immediately placed on a modified MA-1 ventilator. Anyone familiar with normal development would expect a 2-year-old to be rather "negative" in his dealings with others. The "terrible twos", the label often given to the period from 18 months–3 years, is marked by the child's need to have more control over his environment. Most likely he is learning to be toilet trained and is very energetic and curious.

The adult nurse who views all pediatric patients as "children" rather than as 2-year-olds, three-year-olds, etc. might experience problems. For example, this 2-year-old boy would need his mother close by and based on his activity level, might need to be restrained. The nurse should also expect some general regression of behavior such as bedwetting and the need for a bottle for feedings even though the child was previously toilet trained and weaned.

Physiologically, there are also important age-related differences. A 2-year-old would most definitely have a small endotracheal tube in place, perhaps a size 4.0–5.0 internal diameter tube. This would require that the nurse have smaller suction catheters available to ensure patency of the tube. Blood loss from the child's chest tubes need careful monitoring. Any blood loss greater than 2 cc/kg/hr is cause for concern. For example, in a child weighing 16 kg a blood loss of 32 cc/hr is a significant loss. That amount, however, would be insignificant in an adult patient. The use of an adult-size ventilator (MA-1) for a small child would also need careful attention. The small tidal volumes that children require coupled with lower flow rates could lead to problems with ventilating a young child's lungs. Use of small-sized tubings from the machine to the patient and careful monitoring of chest expansion are necessary to ensure adequate ventilation.

The important point made by these examples is that the care and monitoring of children requires special skills just as the care and monitoring of an adult does. It is difficult to mix two very different areas of specialization, pediatric nursing and adult nursing. Each is unique and separate unto itself. Because of the specialized training of each nurse, it would seem logical that patients are best cared for in their own environment. Quality of care for children should be highest when the child is cared for in a pediatric ICU designed for children, equipped with pediatric-sized equipment, and managed by pediatric-trained nurses.

Cost Effectiveness

Cost effectiveness is a timely issue, certainly relevant to this discussion. It is reasonable to assume that pediatric ICUs cannot and are not intended to be set up in every hospital. In fact, the Joint Commission on Accreditation of Hospitals publishes standards that determine which hospitals qualify as centers. Usually a medical school affiliation and geographic accessibility are critical factors in the selection of one hospital over another. Public Law 93-641 advises that health care planning be done through regulating agencies. The intent of the law is that various persons such as health administrators, nurses, and physicians be involved in deciding which hospitals are regional centers and which receive resources. The American Academy of Pediatrics also publishes guidelines for establishment of pediatric ICUs.

Including children in an already existing adult ICU requires a minimal financial commitment. Provided the bed space is available, the acquisition of pediatric equipment may be necessary in some cases. The real cost is in training nurses to care for children. This factor has been bypassed in many cases, and any competent adult nurse is assigned to care for critically ill children. Although not ideal, this situation seems reasonable for a hospital with a limited number of pediatric cases.

Setting up a separate pediatric ICU requires a large financial commitment. Providing the space is available within a general hospital, the exact size of the unit would need to be determined in accordance with projected use. The American Academy of Pediatrics suggests that 10% of the total number of children's beds should be intensive care beds. Specialized equipment and trained personnel including a medical and nursing director, would need to be secured. All support services such as nutrition, respiratory therapy, and laboratories would need to be involved. Needless to say, the costs make setting up a unit prohibitive in many cases.

A viable alternative, especially if no more than five pediatric ICU beds are needed, might be to convert a part of an adult ICU into a pediatric ICU and to provide trained pediatric nurses to care for the children. A limited amount of pediatric equipment would be necessary to ensure appropriate monitoring of critically ill children. This alternative would ensure care of children by nurses with knowledge in growth and development factors as well as critical care concepts. Ideally, the children would be isolated from the adult patients to provide a quieter, less threatening, and more comfortable environment for the children and their families.

Another alternative, in view of rising medical costs, would be to develop regional centers for pediatric critical care. Regionalization of services is not a new idea. Neonatal services have been successfully regionalized and can serve as a model. The idea could be studied by the Joint Commission on Accreditation of Hospitals as well as the American Academy of Pediatrics. Criteria for standards could be established and various sites across the country considered. A transport network could be established such as those for high-risk neonates, to ensure availability of care for even the most remote areas.

Staff Retention

The job satisfaction and retention of the nursing staff in an adult ICU may be affected by the presence of patients who require different routines and have different needs. Critically ill children are often "dumped" in an adult ICU because space is unavailable elsewhere. Adult nurses may resent being assigned to care for children, a situation in which they have little interest in or knowledge about the patient. Likewise, the presence of pediatric nurses in an adult ICU may lead to conflict, because the pediatric nurse will need to adjust to different equipment and a whole different environment, one often lacking in children-oriented accoutrements such as colorful wallpaper, mobiles, and rocking chairs.

In either case, the nurse may be out of the most natural environment. This may create enough tension to lead to job dissatisfaction and thus affect retention.

Educational Needs of Nursing Staff

Overall Needs. All critical care nurses have a great need for educational offerings. Quality educational programs are well-established for adult-oriented critical care nurses. For example, the American Association of Critical-Care Nurses (AACN) annually provides a week-long National Teaching Institute whereby current advances in knowledge and technology across a broad spectrum of topics that include pediatrics and neonatology are provided to help nurses keep abreast of the rapidly changing field. Throughout the year AACN also sponsors numerous 1- and 2-day Regional Teaching Institutes that generally address a specific area. Further, almost 200 local AACN chapters nationwide provide year-long educational programs ranging from monthly evening lectures and hands-on workshops to 1-, 2-, and 3-day symposia. Several international chapters are active, and the first International Teaching Institute will be presented in London in August, 1982. An overwhelming majority of AACN presentations are given by nurse experts whose knowledge, clinical expertise, interest in research, and teaching ability is of the highest caliber. Despite the availability of these and other programs, a dearth of adult critical care textbooks exists (both in nursing and medicine) to help orient and provide advanced information to the nurse.

A special problem exists with respect to pediatric critical care oriented programs; only a limited number of quality offerings are available. One of the primary reasons for this has been the lack of qualified, clinically competent nurses with graduate education to teach advanced pediatric material. Furthermore, the nursing literature in pediatric critical care is scant. In 1981, only two nursing books were in print,[4,5] and these were supplemented by only one medical text.[6]

The outcome is that the chance that adult nurses will attend quality educational programs specific to pediatrics is limited. Furthermore, it may also be unlikely that an adult nurse would have the energy or desire to learn a new specialty relatively unaided. Whereas pediatric nurses are affected by the same program limitations overall, they have a better chance of upgrading their knowledge and skills as more nurses with the master's degree assume positions in pediatric settings. Currently, organizations such as AACN are devoting entire day sessions around the country to pediatric critical care concepts. AACN is also planning to develop a pediatric critical care core curriculum and competency exam to complement its existing adult core curriculum and qualification exam, leading to certification in critical care (CCRN).

Orientation Programs. The usual procedure in educating critical care nurses is to provide an intensive orientation program prior to allowing the nurse to work independently with a critically ill patient. One approach to clinical orientation might be to provide close supervision for each orientee by a specified preceptor. Ideally, the preceptor and orientee are fairly well-matched in style and personality. The clinical orientation should be accompanied by classroom teaching that relates advanced concepts in applied physiology to nursing assessment and intervention. Today, an orientation program consisting solely of on-the-job training is obsolete with respect to the vast realm of current and future critical care nursing.

The orientation program for pediatric critical care nursing must include not only the usual areas of physiology, nursing procedures, and interventions but also the growth and developmental aspects of each area. It is precisely the issues of growth and development that make caring for children especially complicated at times. Programs designed to train the adult-oriented nurse in caring for children should, therefore, include a discussion of the pediatric components in each area of concern to ensure that the nurse has sufficient and appropriate knowledge to be able to care for critically ill children. Pediatric nurses similarly require intensive information specific to the child, but more emphasis should be placed on the differences between various ages of children.

A comprehensive orientation to care for critically ill children should include emphasis on physical assessment, since very obvious differences occur between children and adults. In addition to the major differences in the vital sign parameters between adults and children, common occurrences in children include sinus arrhythmia, bronchovesicular breath sounds, and diaphragmatic breathing. Signs and symptoms of cardiac and respiratory failure also manifest differently in children.

Fluid, electrolyte, and nutritional considerations are of vital importance with a child (see Chapter 4). It is essential that the nurse caring for children knows each child's fluid and caloric needs and how to calculate them. It is common to care for children who are not receiving the appropriate number of calories; this occurs for various reasons. The amount of weight gain or loss in a 24-hr period must be closely monitored. A weight loss or gain of only 30 gms may be significant in a small infant.

Neurologic assessment and care is another important area that needs to be emphasized in an orientation program. Children respond differently to neu-

Table 9-1. Orientee and Preceptor Guidelines*

Orientee Guidelines	Preceptor Guidelines
1. The orientee and preceptor should have the same patient assignment for a period of at least 3 months.	
2. The orientee and preceptor should have the same working days for the 3-month period.	
3. The orientee should review the policies and procedures of the Unit.	3. The preceptor should be well oriented to the policies and procedures of the Unit.
4. The orientee should participate with the preceptor in weekly goal-setting sessions.	4. The preceptor should help the orientee organize work and set priorities— goal–setting should be done for 2 week periods with a weekly review of the goals.
5. The orientee should participate with the preceptor in weekly evaluation of the established goals.	5. The preceptor should offer the orientee weekly feedback as well as follow-through.
6. The orientee should be aware of basic teaching–learning concepts and his/her role as a learner.	6. The preceptor should demonstrate an ability to teach theory with practical application.
7. The orientee should take the initiative in pursuing independent learning.	7. The preceptor should be a level B nurse**
8. The orientee should know and verbally acknowledge his/her limits and know when to seek help.	8. The preceptor should have worked in the Unit for at least 1 year.
9. The orientee should be aware of and support the philosophy of the Unit.	9. The preceptor should be supportive of the philosophy of the Unit.
10. The orientee should be able to organize time effectively to complete the workload on time.	10. The preceptor should be supportive in crisis and willing to give positive reinforcement.

* Adapted from Pediatric Critical Care Orientation Manual, Rush Presbyterian-St. Luke's Medical Center

** Briefly, a Level B nurse is one who has practiced in the unit at least 1 yr. "B" is the second level of a 4 level clinical ladder. The same 4 areas of development (administration, education, clinical and research) apply to each level. The behaviors elicited in these areas become more complex with advancement to level D

Table 9-2. Expectations of a Pediatric Critical Care Nurse*

The Pediatric Critical Care Nurse will

  provide continuing, comprehensive care, and supportive treatment as required to maintain life
    and to aid recovery of acutely ill children.

  provide emotionally supportive care to acutely ill children.

  provide empathetic support to parents and families of children in the ICU.

  act as an integral and essential member of the health-care team by assessing patient needs and
    by planning care and evaluating its effectiveness.

  serve as a nursing care consultant when children who require some intensive nursing care are
    admitted to regular pediatric units.

  act as a child advocate by ensuring that basic human rights are respected.

  serve as a member of appropriate unit committees.

  teach intensive care nursing principles and skills to appropriate groups.

  function effectively and safely, and demonstrate the following capabilities:

    good physical and emotional health to withstand the stress of continually nursing critically ill
      children,

    knowledge of pathophysiology of underlying diseases,

    knowledge and understanding of sophisticated monitoring equipment and special apparatus,

    ability to reason objectively and to judge and be aware of rapidly changing situations

    ability to interpret data and to act rapidly and decisively,

    ability to perform complex technical skills correctly and in an organized manner,

    ability to record data concisely, accurately, and thoroughly,

    understanding of impact of illness on the life of a child,

    understanding of parental response and ways of coping with the stress of a critically ill child.

* Adapted from Pediatric Critical Care Orientation Manual, Rush Presbyterian-St. Luke's
Medical Center

Table 9-3. Skills List*

Respiratory Care	Discussed or Demonstrated	Performance Date	Comments
A. Use of wall oxygen system with setup of: oxygen mask, heated aerosol unit, oxygen tent, T-tube			
B. Use of suction equipment— amount of appropriate suction for age			
C. Manual resuscitation bags— appropriate sizes and use of			
D. Suction Catheters— appropriate sizes of and use of			
E. Oral airways—appropriate sizes and insertion of			
F. Endotracheal tubes— appropriate sizes, taping, cutting and care of			
G. Tracheostomy tubes— appropriate sizes, insertion of, and care of			

* Partial skills list from Pediatric Critical Care Orientation Booklet, Rush Presbyterian-St.
Luke's Medical Center

Table 9-4. Expectations after Orientation*

Category	Activity	Expected Outcomes	Resources

Respiratory Care
Asthma
Epiglottitis
Croup
Foreign body
   obstruction
RDS
BPD
Pulmonary edema
Pneumothorax
Pneumonia
	Reviews anatomy,
	   physiology, clinical
	   manifestations, nursing
	   assessment, and
	   treatment of each
	   disorder
	Reviews signs and
	   symptoms of
	   complications for each
	   disorder and
	   understands the nursing
	   interventions for each
	   complication
	Reviews the medications
	   commonly used in
	   children with
	   respiratory disorders,
	   and the dosage, side
	   effects and interaction
	   effects of each:
	      epinephrine
	      racemic epinephrine
	      isoproterenol
	      aminophylline/
	         theophylline
	      antibiotics
	      steroids
		Assesses respiratory
		   status and
		   interprets
		   complications
		   correctly
		Appropriately
		   monitors patient
		   status with
		   respiratory therapy
		   equipment
		Demonstrates ability
		   to correlate blood
		   gases with
		   patient's status
		Demonstrates ability
		   to administer
		   medications
		   appropriately
		      oral
		      IM
		      IV
		      IV drip
			Respiratory Clinical
			   Specialist
			Respiratory
			   Therapist
			Chest
			   Physiotherapist

* Adapted partial list of expectations from Pediatric Critical Care Orientation Manual, Rush Presbyterian-St. Luke's Medical Center

rologic trauma and exhibit different signs of increased intracranial pressure as compared with adults. Many times the most hopeless-appearing child may rally neurologically and seem to "beat all odds."

Finally, specific attention should be devoted to the appropriate techniques of cardiopulmonary resuscitation in infants and children. Emergency medications are often difficult to use since the dosages are so dependent on body weight of the individual child.

The following discussion of a specific orientation program for pediatric nurses may provide more insight into the necessary depth of information that should be provided for nurses caring for children regardless of the specific kind of unit in which the child is housed.

At Rush Presbyterian–St. Luke's Medical Center in Chicago, the Orientation Committee of the Pediatric Intensive Care Unit is in charge of implementing the program for orientees in the 12-bed unit. Each orientee is paired with a preceptor for a period of not less than 3 months. Specific guidelines are established for both the orientee and preceptor roles (Table 9-1). The expectations of a pediatric critical care nurse are documented in Table 9-2. A 150-page manual that provides specific information regarding expected behaviors of the orientee at the end of the orientation period is given to each orientee. A skills list (Table 9-3) has been established to aid the orientee and preceptor in deciding which skills need to be mastered. All skills are demonstrated first by the preceptor, after which the orientee repeats the demonstration. A space in the manual, to be signed by the preceptor when a skill is successfully demonstrated, provides a permanent record for the orientee.

Table 9-4, Expectations after Orientation, illustrates categories of nursing activities (such as respiratory care), specific care activities related to these categories, expected outcomes, and resources. Orientees are expected to dem-

Table 9-5. Topics for a Pediatric Orientation Program*

Respiratory Care
  Review of anatomy and physiology
  Interpretation of arterial blood gases
  Physical assessment of the child
  Oxygenation
    Oxygen delivery systems
    $TcPO_2$ monitoring
  Chest X-Ray interpretation
  Artificial airways
  Chest tubes
  Chest physiotherapy
  Mechanical ventilation in the infant and the child

Cardiac Care
  Review of anatomy and physiology
  Physical assessment of the child
  Cardiac catheterization/Echocardiogram
  Congenital heart defects
  Surgical repair of congenital heart defects
  Congestive heart failure
  Cardiac drugs
  Pacemakers in children
  Shock
  Measurement of cardiac output

Neurologic Care
  Review of anatomy and physiology
  Physical assessment
  Increased intracranial pressure
  Seizures
  Meningitis
  Reyes syndrome
  Head trauma

Renal Care
  Review of anatomy and physiology
  Physical assessment
  Fluid and electrolyte balance
  Renal failure

General
  Total parenteral nutrition
  DIC
  Burns
  Multiple trauma
  Poisoning

* From Pediatric Critical Care Unit, Rush Presbyterian-St. Luke's Medical Center

onstrate the appropriate proficiencies by the end of 3 months. These guidelines serve as standards for the orientee and as teaching guidelines for the preceptor. In addition, the manual provides information about unit policies besides specific guidelines for care of children with cardiovascular, respiratory, neurologic, gastrointestinal, and renal disorders.

The clinical orientation is augmented by organized classroom teaching. This consists of four weeks of classes (3 sessions/week) in which expert nurses, physicians, and therapists present pediatric-oriented information. Table 9-5 shows the various information presented in the classroom part of the orientation. In addition, all nurses are required to complete a certification course in pediatric chest physiotherapy, a hemodynamic workshop, and a cardiac arrhythmia course within the first 6 months of employment.

At the end of the classroom training, a comprehensive examination is administered to all orientees. The nurse must achieve a passing grade to practice independently in the ICU. After working directly with the orientee, the preceptor evaluates both clinical skills and performance of such skills as coping with a mock arrest and setting up equipment. The 3-month orientation period is extended if either the preceptor or orientee considers that more time is needed to synthesize new information and skills.

Future Trends in Critical Care Pediatrics

The predictions for the future in terms of demographic trends with reference to children lend credence to the need for more sophisticated health care services for children. Two current deficits need to be corrected: more energy must be directed to preventive health care for children, and facilities for comprehensive acute care of children must be established.

The development of the subspecialty of neonatology, established in 1977, can serve as a standard on which pediatric critical care can model itself. In 1980, just three years after the subspecialty was established, there were over 500 certified neonatology medical specialists.[1] In addition, neonatology specialty programs are being offered at the master's level in nursing, thus ensuring that nurses who are involved in neonatal critical care are provided with competent nurse educators who can impart the sophisticated information necessary to work with high-risk neonates.

Establishment of a comprehensive regional system, whereby certain centers nationwide are designated as high-risk centers has been very successful. Neonatal mortality has decreased, and morbidity is decreasing as well. The lack of similiar programs in pediatrics has been disappointing. The health care system must address the special needs of the critically ill child today to be prepared for future trends.

One of the most underdeveloped areas in caring for the critically ill child is the prehospital phase. In 1973, the Emergency Medical Services Act defined an EMS system as one that "provides for the arrangement of personnel, facilities and equipment for the effective and coordinated delivery of health care services under emergency conditions."[7] Very little has been done in this area since that time with regard to children.

The need for nationwide regionalization of pediatric ICUs and the establishment of an EMS specific to pediatrics has been documented.[8] The National Center for Health Statistics shows that in 1976 approximately 21,500 children between the ages of 1–14 years died.[9] Approximately 60% (12,628) of the deaths were attributed to so-called EMS diseases—accidents, poisonings, violence, ischemic heart disease, and acute treatable diseases. If pediatric deaths in children under 1 year of age are included, the annual number of deaths due to emergencies jumps to about 20,000.[10] It is reasonable to assume that an optimal EMS system could have prevented some of these deaths.

Coupled with a pediatric EMS system could be the consolidation of existing pediatric ICUs into centers capable of handling the most acute of cases. These centers should be established across the country and each should be associated with a transport system to ensure availability of care to all children in a designated region.

The idea is not without problems. Because of the small number of patients involved (approximately 195 pediatric EMS fatalities/million population/year compared with approximately 3810 EMS-related deaths/year in adults),[9] the program will not be cost effective at first in terms of training personnel and providing continuing education, etc. The pediatric component of the EMS system should complement the already established adult system. A uniform communications system needs to be developed. Thus far most transport equipment, such as defibrillators are not tailored for children's needs; this deficiency needs to be remedied.

Finally, regional cooperation in the planning of an EMS system for children is necessary. More rural areas should be considered and personnel educated to participate in the planning and implementation phases.

A model for a pediatric transport system does exist in Denver.[10] Developed in 1979, a 500,000-square-mile region is served by the Denver Pediatric Emergency Transportation system. A flexible air–ground transport system serves the rural and mountain areas as well as the high-density metropolitan region. Three designated hospitals provide comprehensive care once the children are transported.

A similar system needs to be developed across the nation. Standards need to be set and regional centers identified. This requires the support of the Federal Government, agencies such as the American Heart Association, American Lung Association, American Association of Critical-Care Nurses, physicians, and nurses. In the long run, such a regional program should decrease morbidity as well as mortality, thus reducing the number of hospital days, the requirement for nursing care, and rehabilitation time.

Such an endeavor also requires a comprehensive orientation and educational program for nurses. The program should include the principles and practice of transporting critically ill children, which encompasses the methods and problems of transporting and the process of stabilizing the children once they reach the hospital. Pediatric intensivists and nurses should become actively involved in local and national planning through their professional organizations and communities. Standards need to be developed for care-giver roles, responsibilities and educational needs, and for educational programs. As a corollary, pediatric critical care nursing and medical literature needs to be developed.

The prospect of a regionalized system for transport and care of critically ill children is exciting. The only way for pediatric medicine and nursing to be viable in the care of critically ill children is to begin work today.

REFERENCES

1. Holbrook P: The scope of pediatric critical care. Crit Care Med 8:535, 1980
2. Selim R: Health in the future: in the pink or in the red. The Futurist 8:329, 1979
3. Fagin C, Nusbaum J: Parental visiting privileges in pediatric units: a survey. J Nurs Adm 8:25, 1978
4. Vestal K: Pediatric Critical Care Nursing. New York, Wiley Med Pub, 1981
5. American Association of Critical-Care Nurses: Critical Care Nursing of Children and Adolescents. ed. Oakes AR. New York, Saunders, 1981
6. Levin D: A Practical Guide to Pediatric Intensive Care. St Louis, CV Mosby, 1979
7. Public Law 93-154: Emergency Medical Services System Act of 1973, November 16, 1973
8. National Research Council Committee on Trauma: Accidental Death and Disability: the Neglected Disease of Modern Society. Washington DC, National Academy of Sciences, 1966
9. Vital Statistics Report, Final Mortality Statistics, 1976. National Center for Health Statistics, Department of Health, Education and Welfare publication no 78-1120, vol 26, 12, suppl (2), March 30, 1978
10. Dobrin R, Block B, Gilman J, Massaro T: The development of a pediatric emergency transport system. Pediatr Clin North Am 27:633, 1980

10 | Management of the Primary Nursing Model in the Pediatric Critical Care Unit

Eileen Pierce

The ultimate goal of nursing within any critical care setting is to deliver quality care to the patient. Methods of delivery vary from institution to institution and in many instances are directly related to staff composition. Variations in method range from functional nursing, team nursing, and case method to primary nursing. One of the critical ingredients in the decision regarding which method to use is the accountability necessary for quality care.

The many technologic advances in critical care nursing do not make the job easier but rather require patient care to be more exact. Consequently, there is an everpresent need for more interpretation, which requires a method of care that is not fragmented. Each medication, treatment, fluid requirement intervention and their total effect have paramount importance on the well-being of the patients and require the expertise of nurses prepared to be accountable for the delivery of total patient care.

In the Pediatric Critical Care Unit (PCCU) a variety of complex situations of care present themselves in a very delicate balance. It is necessary to identify one knowledgeable professional nurse for the patient and family to preserve the physical, developmental, emotional and social balance of the child and family.

Much of the literature has described a method of care delivery through a primary nursing system. This philosophy of care responds to the needs of the nurse and the patient as well. The method of primary nursing provides for accountability, advocacy for the patient, and autonomy for the nurse.[1]

Success of this method in any institution requires strong support from within the system. The system assumes a different working relationship among nurses who are now referred to as primary and associate nurses and with the head nurse/unit leaders who assume management responsibilities for success of the system at the unit level. Each individually assumes a new dimension in role expectations from the traditional roles.[2]

In the following sections primary nursing in the PCCU will be addressed. Specific areas that will be discussed more fully are accountability, role changes, potential hazards within the primary nursing system, and communication within such a structure.

PRIMARY NURSING MEETING THE NEEDS OF THE NURSES

That nurses should return to the patient's bedside is not only the cry of a demanding society but also that of a new breed of nurses who insist upon practicing what they once learned in school. Men and women in the profession of nursing are embarking on an era of challenge and change. The front runners of the era will be those who are willing to test their clinical competence and lay the foundation for more responsibility and greater accountability.

With each passing day nurses are becoming more cognizant of their new and more significant role, standing side-by-side with, yet apart from physicians in planning and delivering care to their patients. The manner in which nursing expresses the relative autonomy of this new role is realized through an organizational structure that fosters parity with the physician.

As the major planner and giver of care at the bedside of a critically ill patient, a nurse is not only an observer and deliverer of care, as suggested by the physician, but also the assessor, planner, and teacher for both the patient and family through "discharge planning," which begins on the day of admission and defines Primary Nursing.[3]

Through careful orchestration of the primary nursing system, the professional nurse is able to undertake a new challenge in the form of planning and interpreting a patient's response to treatments. The totality of care required of the nurse provides for a degree of control over the planning for and evaluation of care received by his/her patient caseload. Additionally, it allows nurses to be creative, accountable, and cognizant of the care of their primary patients from admission through discharge, attributes that elude the nurse practicing in a more traditional setting.

PRIMARY NURSING CAN PROVIDE WHAT THE CHILD AND FAMILY NEED

"Development does not stop at birth, important developmental changes, in addition to (cellular) growth, occur after birth. Most developmental changes are completed by the age of 25." From this statement made by Keith L. Moore in *The Developing Human,*[4] one might observe that a child is an unparalleled being, in a state of constant change and equipped with all the 'potential' to be an adult. Potential, however, is that which is possible but not yet actualized.

The physical, emotional, and developmental aspects of childhood that lead to adulthood require nurturing and interpretation. Growth in each of these areas proceeds normally where there is health and security. However, when health is interrupted, the normal cellular growth and emotional and developmental security are also disturbed. In the face of illness requirements for growth become more in need of delicate mediating to regain their delicate balance.

A child's ability to interpret his own world and to express his needs and desires grows steadily in a secure, healthy world. Conventional modes of communication that are taken for granted in an adult world do not totally exist at the various levels of a child's development. Language is also an important consideration as an adult attempts to gain trust and render an explanation to a child. The explanations must fit the child's chronologic and developmental age. Identifying the child's level of understanding, mode of communication, and ability to cope all become important tools in preserving his level of development and gaining his trust and eventually his cooperation. In our society parents have been entrusted with the enormous responsibility of balance, interpretation, and guidance for total child development. But what becomes of the delicate balance when a child is removed from his home because his health has been interrupted? Who provides for his needs in the hospital environment that is so foreign and outside the realm of control for both the child and his family?

The primary nurse has been defined in the literature as the one specific person designated as responsible for planning and giving care in a hospital setting. In pediatric critical care this singularity in the provision of care seems especially logical when one considers that the most significant responsible person in a child's life is referred to as the primary care giver.[5] We cannot assume from this a replacement of the primary care giver but rather an extension of that role in an environment that necessitates the addition of so many sophisticated and technical responsibilities. The totality of needs in the developing, growing individual permits and perhaps demands the philosophy of primary nursing. For this reason caring for a critically ill child is a unique and awesome responsibility. The nurse becomes entrusted with the responsibility of physical care, emotional and developmental nurturing, education, and support of the child.

In addition to the child's needs, the needs of the family must be addressed. Their needs will vary with their own maturity. Many families have no knowledge of a hospital critical care unit; many have never experienced the death of a loved one; and many are parents for the first time. They all, however, are experiencing a common catastrophy—their child's illness.

Society-at-large is both unfamiliar and uncomfortable with catastrophic disease or death of a child. Therefore, families are often left unsupported during these difficult times by a caring but perhaps ill-prepared extended family or group of friends. The family support area of nursing, then, becomes as necessary as the care of the ill child himself.

INTERRELATIONSHIPS AMONG INDIVIDUALS
AND GROUPS

In primary nursing an assumption exists for accountability to the client, to the macrosystem, to the microsystem, and to their relative interrelationships.

The word *accountability* must be defined and keenly supported for the successful application of an organizational structure such as primary nursing. The word is at times over-used and will lose meaning unless it is allowed to evolve. The definition of accountability for our purposes can be derived from two sources. One source is Webster's dictionary which states: "Accountability is responsibility for a trust."[6] The second source is the definition used by Natalie Petzold in the book entitled *Accountability: A Challenge to Educators,* in which she described accountability as "that which deals with the rights and responsibilities, the 'answer-abilities' or liabilities of individuals and of groups and the interrelationships among them."[7]

Beginning with the macro structure—the level above the patient-care unit—accountability is assumed by hospital administrators whose energies are devoted to the support services essential to the smooth operations of primary nursing. It is best when the non-nursing functions traditionally relegated to nursing can be assumed by other persons.[8] Tasks such as answering the telephone, doing housekeeping chores, and transporting patient specimens remove nurses further from the bedside. These tasks now fall into more appropriate hands. Hospital administration therefore assumes a "responsibility for a trust." The road toward primary nursing becomes facilitated and nursing is removed from a vacuum.

Accountability is assumed by nursing administrators through support to their constituents in the form of budgeted staff positions as well as educational and managerial support. It is the nursing administration acting in conjunction with hospital administration that conceived the idea for and are entrusted with the responsibility for maintaining the necessary atmosphere for primary nursing within the institution.

A second level of accountability is the microsystem (the unit) and its responsibility to the nurse. How does one assist a nurse at the unit level to become accountable? The person who directs the development of staff accountability at the unit level has traditionally been referred to as a head nurse/ unit leader. Indeed, the management of the process of change from a team/ functional system to a primary nursing system is a delicate task that falls most heavily on the head nurse/unit leader.[9] The part this individual plays in the success or failure of the primary nursing system on the unit cannot be underestimated.

In the past it was the head nurse/unit leader who was responsible and recognized to be the most knowledgeable person on the unit regarding the current status of each patient. It was the head nurse/unit leader who was respectfully sought for by everyone and who was responsible for accompanying the physician on rounds and communicating with him regarding the patient's condition and the plan of care for the remaining 24 hrs. The head nurse/unit leader might outline the care on a designated kardex, and the staff in turn would follow this written prescribed treatment plan. This method stripped the staff nurse not only of planning responsibilities but also of recognition, creativity, thinking, and individualizing techniques of patient care. The staff nurse within such a structure remained an anonymous worker. Nursing practices in these instances helped to breed both apathy and atrophy and divested the staff nurse of accountability.

In order for the necessary change of accountability for direct patient care to take place as prescribed by a primary nursing system, the individual who assumes the title of head nurse/unit leader must be assured of support of the nursing administration during the transition from 'doer and knower of all' with her hand maidens to organizer and planner in a more global sense. Because responsibility and recognition for patient care changes hands, the head nurse/ unit leader may feel threatened and relieved of authority.

The direction that middle management assumes is expressed in a new dimension within a primary nursing setting. Areas that were untouched and untested by this level of management become the arena for the head nurse/ unit leaders. Areas such as budgeting, interviewing, hiring, terminating employment, disciplining, assessing unit needs, and the ever-important areas of role modeling and planning for unit development become the tools of their now more global role.

Others—for example, the physicians—who have grown in the traditional setting of nursing practice, also receive their reinforcement for behavior change from the head nurse/unit leader. The role transition demands the time and patience of everyone concerned. The head nurse/unit leader may need to introduce a physician to his/her patient's primary nurse several times in one day. Eventually, however, the transition will occur and will be evidenced to all when any person comes to the PCCU and requests to speak with a particular patient's primary nurse to discuss the patient's progress and plan for his discharge.

ACCOUNTABILITY EVOLVES THROUGH PARTICIPATION

Accountability cannot be presumed on graduation from nursing school. Yet to practice primary nursing one agrees to 24-hr accountability—24 hrs of "responsibility for a trust." To assist in the growth toward accountability becomes the charge of the system within which primary nursing is practiced.

The first step in developing the concept of 24-hr accountability may be to allow nurses to participate in the determination of primary nursing, which can be accomplished by a participative management technique. Surveying the staff nurses for both their philosophy of family-centered care and their objectives for primary nursing fosters their developing expectations of themselves within a primary nursing structure in a PCCU.

Behavior expressed in action should be prefaced by thoroughly conceived written objectives formed by the staff assuming the new philosophy. Through this participative management technique, each staff nurse may realize the important role his/her individuality plays in the process of patient care. In addition a "team effort" that becomes the foundation for critical care nursing is formulated. An example, developed by the PCCU of the Rush-Presbyterian-St. Luke's Medical Center in Chicago, is given below.

PHILOSOPHY AND OBJECTIVES DEVELOPED THROUGH STAFF PARTICIPATION

Philosophy, Pediatric Critical Care Unit

Because a child is a unique person dependent upon the world about him for meeting his needs, we realize the interdependence of the child-family-nurse.

Because disease interrupts the multi-faceted psycho-social life, and physical integrity of a child and family, we realize the need for emphathy, education, support, and service.

Because hospitalization is a traumatic experience for the family unit, we realize the possibility of regression and recognize our obligation to maintain the family's ability to deal with stress.

Because of the specialization of the Pediatric Critical Care Unit, the equipment involved, and the need for constant monitoring, we realize the obligation of staff to teach and constantly reinforce to the patient and the family the rationale behind the need for specific kinds of care and treatments.

Because of the need for specialized technical care and interpersonal aspects of care, we realize the need for staff education, communication, and personal development.

Because we are a part of a University Medical Center, we realize our obligation to be role models, professionally and technically, to nursing and medical students.

Objectives, Pediatric Critical Care Unit

1. To identify the growth and developmental level of functioning for each patient

2. To identify the specific criteria and assessment tools needed for evaluating and monitoring each bodily function through the use of specialized equipment.

3. To provide an orientation period prior to the patient's admission to the Pediatric Critical Care Unit to alleviate anxiety and elicit cooperation.

4. To coordinate the various methods of treatment with the developmental age and level of functioning of each patient.

5. To recognize the patient-family relationship and present their interdependence in a working care plan.

6. To identify the troubled communications of patient and family in interpersonal relationships and to follow through with further recommendations for appropriate consultations prior to and after discharge.

7. To educate patient and family to health maintenance and disease prevention.

8. To assist patient and family in accepting the outcomes of any disease process or debilitation.

9. To provide an atmosphere for rehabilitation through appropriate referrals.

10. To provide a stimulating, professional, and intense educational opportunity for nursing and medical staffs.

11. To continuously maintain open channels of communication between nurse, physician, and others involved in delivering care.

12. To provide continuity of care through the development of current care plans and patient care conferences.

ACCOUNTABILITY PRESUMES KNOWLEDGE

Primary nursing demands a high level of decision making skill in addition to skills needed in clinical nursing—i.e., planning, assessing, and evaluating the condition of the patient. Pediatric critical care nursing necessitates a separate body of knowledge from that needed in adult critical care nursing. The primary nursing system continues to prepare a nurse for a 24-hr "accountability for a trust" through education. Education must be a continual process beginning with orientation. Orientation sessions are required to address not only the physical conditions that will be encountered and the required assessment and mechanical skills but also growth and development of a child, stress management, dealing with death, and a review of expectations of a critical care nurse. Through such a program a level of staff competence can be assured, a level that will assist in fostering responsibility for a trust between the primary nurse and associate nurse, the primary nurse and physician, and the primary nurse and client.

Through a complete understanding of and practice in administering general pediatric care as well as competence in techniques of critical care nursing and crisis intervention, the pediatric critical care nurse begins to incorporate assessment techniques that differ from those of adult nursing. For example, medication dosages and fluid requirements that are similar for most adult patients become minute dosages that must be individualized according to the ever-changing weight of the child. In addition there is a dramatic difference in the attention to detail that is required in caring for adults compared with caring for children. The consequences to an adult patient who is NPO for several hours without intravenous feeding are minimal when compared with the catastrophic consequences to a 10-lb infant who is NPO without intravenous feeding for the same period of time. Relatively large amounts of blood may be taken from adults without harmful results; whereas in children the volume of blood taken for tests must be strictly accounted for, since even relatively small losses need replacement.

In addition to the vastly different physical requirements in adults and children, a working knowledge and understanding of normal growth and development, and an understanding of the needs of families in crisis, the nurse becomes prepared to assume the role of a primary nurse in a PCCU.

Growth in accountability does not end with orientation. Because critical care technology changes daily, a mechanism must be developed to assure staff members that their knowledge is constantly updated. Staff input into this area of development, not only encourages them to identify the knowledge they need but also builds upon the concept of accountability. Further education may take the form of journal clubs, patient care conferences and in-services presented by the staff for the staff. Through an ongoing educational program the primary nurse is assured of the tools necessary to assume 24-hr accountability. The trust necessary for accountability is strengthened through practice and education.

ACCOUNTABILITY THROUGH DELEGATION

Accountability can be nurtured further through a management technique called "project delegation." Each critical care unit has a variety of projects that need constant review—a systematic evaluation. Among these projects are a primary nurse audit, staff orientation and staff development, policy and procedure review, child–family education, and emergency preparedness, to name just a few. Each of these areas requires staff involvement at the implementation phase. Why not then require the staff also to be involved in the planning stages? A staff nurse who assumes all inclusive responsibility for primary nursing can benefit immeasurably from committee work participation for several reasons.

First, the nurse can change pace for a while, from the stress of patient care responsibility to a less stressful, idea-sharing, idea-testing role. Second, it allows nurses more control over the kinds of tasks for which they will be responsible. Third, it fosters team work on a different level. It requires that individuals meet deadlines for the good of the group. It allows a "practice field" for decision-making. Finally, it previews organizational bureaucracy for certain committees and consequently teaches patience and reality orientation.

An example of the manner in which a staff committee encourages problem-solving, answerability, trust, cooperation, and outcome planning may be seen in the tool that was developed by PCCU staff at Rush-Presbyterian-St. Luke's Medical Center in Chicago (Fig. 10-1). The staff members that have been given an opportunity to define expectations of primary nursing within the PCCU are now able to evaluate the behaviors that they identified as their responsibilities.

With a tool designed by the staff *for the staff*, the audits are performed by the committee members on every 3rd patient admitted to the unit. The audit is brief enough for consistent use in a busy area but provides enough data for determining the effectiveness of the primary nursing system. Through a feed-back mechanism to all staff—a notebook of minutes and unit meeting committee reports—areas that are pinpointed by the audit as needing more staff attention become apparent. In this manner the staff becomes accountable for the process of primary nursing.

The amount of actual authority each committee is given must be predetermined and the committee's charges must be defined. This sets the tone for the committee as to whether to prepare recommendations or to set policy. Nurses serving on the committees are adult men and women and must be recognized as such. Although they may require guidance in the protocols of committee work in a particular institution, they possess all the rights and privileges of adults with ideas. This statement may seem harsh, but isn't it the cry of the professional nurses today that they are not respected? We are often tempted to charge the physician for lack of respect for the nurse; but can we be so certain that various levels of nursing have respect for their own profes-

Primary Nursing Audit Tool

Name:		Date:	YES	NO
1.	Nursing Admissions Record Complete.			
2.	Kardex Complete.			
3.	Admission Soap Note			
	a. Biological			
	b. Behavioral			
	c. Nursing History			
4.	Primary Nurse Identified (24 hours)			
5.	Care Plan			
	a. Problem list			
	b. Expected Outcomes			
	c. Target Dates			
	d. Nursing Interventions			
	e. Identifies Times			
6.	Behavioral Considerations			
7.	Family Considerations			
8.	Inter-Disciplinary			
9.	Evaluation/Revisions			
10.	Discharge Planning			
11.	Patient Care Conference			
Comments:				

Fig. 10-1. Primary nursing audit tool. A tool used for auditing the mechanics of the Primary Nursing system. A separate audit is performed for completeness and quality of the nursing care plan during staff level evaluations. (From the Pediatric Critical Care Unit, Rush-Presbyterian-St. Luke's Medical Center, Chicago, IL.)

sionals? Therein may lay what can be referred to as the "hazards of primary nursing."

The Hazards of Primary Nursing

That primary nursing in its most sophisticated form seems to be the best alternative to quality patient care in a PCCU is difficult to dispute. What then, if anything, may be identified as difficulties or potential hazards of primary nursing? Do the benefits outweigh these difficulties? Finally, is it possible to temper the hazards to best serve the patient, the staff, and the system?

The questions are not easily answered. At times, the obstacles to complete primary nursing may seem too large. The accountability required of each individual at each level within the PCCU increases through this organizational structure of primary nursing. Yet reports in the literature seem to identify a high level of nurse satisfaction with primary nursing.[1] What are the hazards that one might encounter?

"Burnout" Through System Failure

"Burnout" is one of the most frequently talked-about reasons that nurses leave pediatric critical care nursing. It is inappropriate to associate the cause of burnout with primary nursing. However, there is reason to look into the role the primary nursing organizational structure may play on staff burnout if not properly supported.

Burnout is a term that is frequently used today to describe the phenomenon felt by a nurse who has invested in a profession that has consumed him/her. Whether the nurse who practices within a primary nursing system is more susceptible to burnout is questionable. The question, however, may more correctly be asked of the system than of the philosophy.

A variety of factors seem to drive nurses away from critical care or to burn them out. Among these is the mute promise of parity with the physician or at least recognition for the knowledge the nurse possesses. As the essential members of a team effort for the delivery of quality patient care, the primary nurse and physician must assume a close working relationship. Without the exchange of information between them, patient care suffers. The burden for such an exchange falls on each primary nurse and each physician individually. Lack of support for this team approach or the lack of recognition for the information exchange thwarts the efforts of the primary nursing philosophy and adds immeasurably to nursing burnout.

In addition to lack of recognition, burnout seems to occur in critical care units which are short of staff. The lack of sufficient professional nursing staff burdens the existing staff with high workloads and/or with temporary float or agency personnel. Both of these frustrate the philosophy of the primary nursing model. Consequently, quality patient care is more overwhelming in an era of acute nursing shortage, and practicing nursing the way it was meant to be practiced in critical care units becomes more difficult. Therefore, short staffing causes burnout.

Burnout also occurs because the threat of patient loss is ever present to the critical care unit staff. This loss may be devastating to the primary nurse. To devote the tools of assessing, planning, coordinating, and nurturing to a child who is critically ill and is, perhaps, on the doorstep of death, and to the family consumes physical, emotional, and psychologic energy of great intensity. Preserving the staff nurses' feeling of self-worth and their emotional and physical well-being take on paramount importance. It is this stress of loss that contributes to burnout.

Environmental stress itself must be addressed as a possible cause of burnout. The setting is one of crisis orientation. Few things are predictable. The physical floor plan is generally one of total visibility. Sensory stimuli are purposely made to be alarming to the nurses senses. There is often little control over what happens or when it will happen. Sources of support such as laboratories, pharmacy, clerical services, X-ray, physicians, and peers often seem to be less than perfect in the eyes of the staff nurse in either their delivery of a product or approach to particular problems. Value conflicts and moral and ethical issues raise serious questions. The nurse is expected to deal with patients and families in crisis for prolonged hours each day. The list goes on. The total picture of pediatric critical care nursing presents most emphatically the factors necessary for burnout. Primary nursing as a philosophy of care when supported by the micro- and macrosystems may be an answer rather than a potential hazard for at least some of the issues causing resultant burnout—namely lack of recognition, lack of parity and lack of communication.

Combatting Burnout Through Primary Nursing

Recognition of the nurse is considered in a variety of ways; it pertains to nurses as individuals. Factors that contribute to recognition are job flexibility and rewards. Each is necessary and each must have its place. We ask flexibility of a primary nurse in each patient's plan of care, in the scheduled hours of work expected of the nurse, and in overtime. Does the system also allow for flexibility when it is requested by the nurse? Do we allow for mental health or vacation days other than when they are requested weeks in advance? Do we add an element of predictability for the nurse by scheduling rotation patterns 6 months in advance? Do we adhere to traditional 8-hr scheduling patterns, or do we break from tradition and examine ten- or 12-hr patterns? Do we reward the nurse who has been in the system for 2 or 3 or 5 years with fewer rotations to the least popular shifts? Do we reward the nurse who has provided excellence in patient care by commendations or promotions? Do we educate physicians to this collegeal method of delivery of care? Do we allow for library days so that the staff nurse can prepare an inservice or a patient care conference?

All of these questions merely serve to raise our consciousness to the role the system plays in burnout. It also serves, perhaps, to remove primary nursing as a philosophy from the list of "hazards" and encourages us to focus on the system failure.

COMMUNICATION COMBATS BURNOUT IN A
PRIMARY NURSING SYSTEM

Communication as a method of preventing burnout must occur on all levels. Indeed, good communication patterns become the foundation for success in primary nursing. Lack of communication frustrates the attempts at excellence in patient care.

Problems will remain problems until the appropriate people know the details with supporting data. Unless the hospital administration is aware of problems with particular support services, the same problems will continue. Unless the nursing administration is aware of increased workloads, the difficulty in providing staff with necessary tools to practice, and the difficulty in solving unit problems, the unit members will continue to be frustrated in their attempts to practice primary nursing. Unless the medical director is aware of specific patient–family or medical support problems, nurses will continue to be frustrated in their attempts to practice quality care through primary nursing. Unless nurses begin to confront each other with both positive reinforcement and constructive criticism, we will drown ourselves in frustration.

The question then becomes one of how and where should such communication occur. First and foremost it should be an expectation expressed on every level within the hospital. The lines of communication and chain of command should be clearly understood by each member of the PCCU staff. The grievance route should be clear. Through such mechanisms, few problems ever stand a chance of being "lost in the system."

Unit Staff Meetings Provide
Communication

The forums for communication should be consistent and open. Nursing–Medical staff meetings should be held on a frequent basis. The agenda for such meetings might include problem identification, information sharing, committee reports, recognition of jobs well done, and discussion of short-term goals. The meeting place that perhaps provides the best atmosphere for such a meeting should be somewhere away from the unit itself. In some hospitals, the staff meetings are held twice, and each time in the cafeteria meeting room where staff can participate in the discussions while enjoying a cup of coffee. Posting an agenda prior to the meeting day ensures that staff will assume responsibility to consider the agenda item. Placing a definite time limit on the meeting encourages adherence to the agenda so that business can proceed efficiently in a busy unit.

Interaction between Nursing and
Medical Administration

Close working relationships via open communication must exist between the unit's medical director, unit administration, and the unit leadership group. It is this triad that becomes responsible for department-to-department communication at the unit level and planning for long-term projects. New programs, new protocols, and the redefining of individual roles and commitments occur with such shared communication at the unit level.

Staff-Leadership Communication

Encouraging communication by the staff may be difficult. In a unit with staff members of diverse backgrounds and experience and educational levels, developing effective communication patterns takes time. Providing an atmosphere of openness at the unit leadership level may serve as a method of role modeling. Unit leadership has the responsibility consistently to acknowledge excellence in nursing interventions and to discuss difficulties in delivery of nursing care with individual nurses. In such a manner, the staff begins to trust that leadership is genuinely concerned not only with recognizing successes but also with identifying problems. Providing this atmosphere of professional openness can be another important link to decreasing burnout. The atmosphere may invite exploration of intense conflicts within each staff member. Discussions may occur informally regarding such questions as "What did I do wrong?" or "What should I have done differently?" when a nurse new to the unit experiences the death of a child for the first time. Support during such traumatic events may occur with any member of the unit staff if there is an atmosphere of support and sharing. Every attempt should be made to ensure a forum for this type of informal questioning. The forum may be nursing rounds, peer-to-peer consultation, discussions over coffee in the staff cafeteria, or casual conversation in the campus lounge. While not every question will have an answer, no question should go without discussion. The mere recognition of another's query offers boundless support, and attempts to reduce stress of the staff through open communication.

Staff Communication as a Group

After exploration of the need for open communication on a direct, one-to-one basis, it is necessary to focus more clearly on communication patterns of the staff as a group. The position in which this staff find themselves is virtually unparalleled elsewhere in the unit structure. They, perhaps more so than anyone else, are on the front line in maintaining the primary nursing philosophy. The unit—through overtones of emergency, its fishbowl existence, the absolute necessity for a team effort, and its unpredictability—is volatile. The unit staff group needs another kind of communication tool. Although "talking it out" is perhaps the single most effective tool in attempting to reduce stress, it is not any easy tool to perfect. We expect primary nurses to be conversant with children, families, physicians, peers, and others who assist in the care of the child. They in turn need to practice with each other in a controlled setting. Few persons are taught effective communication skills in school or in early family life. Yet, we expect the primary nurse to know all the right words and to be comfortable saying them to anyone as the occasion arises.

Weekly or biweekly meetings with an objective, trained individual in a neutral setting, provide staff with a forum for discussion of their problems as *they* perceive them. It is important that the meetings be voluntary and that unit leadership is in support of the meetings. These discussion groups as stated by Donald Hay and Donald Oken in "The Psychological Stresses of Intensive Care Unit Nursing"[10] provides:

> (a) an avenue for ventilating suppressed intragroup hostilities as well as shared gripes; (b) a recognition that fears, doubts, guilt, and uncertainty are shared acceptable feelings; (c) the abreaction and working through of feelings aroused at times of stress but which cannot be expressed due to work demands; (d) the sharing of innovative ad hoc techniques which individuals have found helpful in dealing with problems arising on the job; (e) recognition of superior abilities and their delineation from masochistic fantasies of omnipotence; (f) a realization that minor mistakes are ubiquitous and inevitable, leading to detoxification of guilt and shame, and (g) the development of constructive solutions for problems and effective suggestions for communication to administration

Through such meetings, problems can become verbalized and resolutions or at least peer support can be generated. This exploration of each aspect of the work experience may turn a potential negative stress that causes burnout into eustress. *"Through it, our aim,"* as stated by Hans Seyle, *"becomes to learn how to recognize our typical response to stress and then to try to modulate our lives in accordance with it."* [11]

Not all stresses felt by the staff will be effectively dealt with in group sessions. Nevertheless, through discussions and perception clarification a process of "individual responsibility for a trust" of sharing and problem-solving by each staff nurse to each other member of the medical team will be initiated.

Written Communication

Another type of communication that is not frequently used has been found to assist individuals to cope with their feelings and decrease stress. Nurses who care for the children who die in pediatric critical care units may need to culminate the relationship that has been formed by the child–family and primary associate nurse. The method or event that has been found to be beneficial is a Memorial Service, planned and written by the critical care unit staff.

Through planning and writing for the service, each person is given an opportunity to remember the children he/she tried to help. Some children they will have known for only a very short time, others for many months. Encouraging staff to express their feelings in a written poem or verse—yet another manner of communication—provides an acceptable outlet for grief and object loss. It also provides an opportunity for the primary nurse to reflect and reaffirm a commitment to this demanding area of pediatric nursing. Two examples of such writings are given below.

THANK YOU MY FRIEND, MY PEER

Today a baby died.

For eight hours I watched as a life passed by.
People all around, hustle, bustle, and yet there I stood with feelings
    of helplessness, sadness, anger, isolation.
What can I say to parents keeping a quiet vigil—waiting, praying,
    hoping.
And, yet, just yesterday we all shared a day of happiness, relief,
    encouragement.

Is there any appropriate response to make when one parent turns to
    you and says "The doctor said there is no hope."
In quiet desperation I can ony stand and be—hold their hand.
Then the last hour passes.
"Two-forty-five" the physician says, and the room is vacated.

Now nothing but the sounds of silence can be heard.
Everyone is gone. Everyone, it seems, except me and a tiny body.
Now the pain begins. Will I ever feel comfortable charging
    medications and equipment to parents who leave here with no
    child?
Will I ever be able to 'prepare a body' without trying to drive my
    thoughts a hundred miles away, trying not to relive the last
    several hours?
Will I ever understand?
Can I ever accept?

Everything's over. And yet, when I'm able to look further than
    myself, someone is there. Someone who hasn't spoken, perhaps,
    but who I know understands. Then I feel warm again.

Thank you, my friend, my peer.

Author, Eileen Pierce, R.N.–1973.

NANCY'S POEM

Look around you,
you will see
a child dying hopelessly.

Look beside him,
faithfully, his family is waiting,
mournfully.

Look once more,
there's you and me
working, watching,
helplessly.

The grief, the loss
affects us too,
we need support
to see us through.

Look again,
your friends are here,
to scream or pray with,
to shed a tear.

We remember well
the children gone,
but our obligations
keep us going on.

For look one more time
and you will see
a child—reaching
hopefully.

Author, Nancy Stanish, R.N.–1980.

CONCLUSION

The philosophy of primary nursing provides for the needs of patients, families and staff. Such a philosophy of care requires step-by-step development and support within each level of an institution. Without this support, primary nursing as a philosophy of care will breed burnout.

The practice of primary nursing presumes accountability. Individuals and groups must be developed in assuming accountability.

The responsibility for developing accountability rests within the ranks of nursing itself. In each case, communication is the foundation for accountability.

Without communication nursing continues to function in a vacuum, and any attempts at primary nursing will be frustrated.

REFERENCES

1. Ciske K: An organization that promotes professional practice. J Nurs Adm 4:28, 1974
2. Marram G, et al: Cost Effectiveness of Primary and Team Nursing. Wakefield, Contemporary Publ, 1976
3. Fairbanks J: Primary nursing: what's so exciting about it. Nursing 80 10:54, 1980
4. Moore KL: Introduction-developmental terms and concepts. In: The Developing Human. Philadelphia, WB Saunders, 1977
5. Zander KS: Primary Nursing: Development and Management. Germantown, An Aspen Publication, 1980
6. Webster N: The Living Webster Encyclopedia Dictionary of the English Language. Chicago, The English Language Institute of America, 1971
7. Petzold N: Introduction. In: Accountability—A Challenge to Educators. New York, National League for Nursing, 1975
8. Elpern EN: Structural and organizational supports for primary nursing. Nurs Clin North Am 12:205, 1977
9. Hegyvary ST: Foundations of primary nursing. Nurs Clin North Am 12:187, 1977
10. Hay D, Oken D: The psychological stresses of intensive care unit nursing. Psychosom Med 34:109, 1972
11. Selye H: On the real benefits of eustress. Psychol Today, 11:(60)–1, 1978

BIBLIOGRAPHY

Adler DC, Shoemaker NJ: AACN Organization and Management of Critical Care Facilities. St Louis, CV Mosby, 1979

Bakke K: Primary nursing: perceptions of a staff. Am J Nurs 74:1432, 1974

Burns D: Feeling Good: The New Mood Therapy. New York, The New American Library, 1981

Druker P: Managing the knowledge worker. The Wall Street Journal, Dow Jones and Company, 1975

Frieberg KH: How parents react when their child is hospitalized. Am J Nurs 72:1270, 1972

Freud A: The role of bodily illness in the mental life of children. Psychoanal Study Child 7:69, 1952

Gyulay JE: Care of the dying child. Nurs Clin North Am 1:11, 1976

Hedenkamp EA: Humanizing the intensive care unit for children. Crit Care Q 3:63, 1980

Jacobsen SP: Stressful situations for neonatal intensive care nurses. Am J Matern Child Nurs 3:144, 1978

Jacox AK: Who defines and controls nursing practice? Am J Nurs 69:977, 1969

Logsdon A: Why primary nursing? Nurs Clin North Am 8:283, 1973

Maas M: Nurse autonomy reality not rhetoric. Am J Nurs 75:2201, 1975

McCarthy D: Primary nursing—its implementation and six month outcome. J Nurs Adm 8:29, 1978

Norris CM: Restlessness: A nursing phenomenon in search of meaning. Nurs Outlook, 23:103, 1975

Page M: Primary nursing: perceptions of a nurse. Am J Nurs 74:1435, 1974

Petrillo M: Preventing hospital trauma in pediatric patients. Am J Nurs 6:1469, 1968

Schmalenberg CE, Kramer M: Dreams and reality: where do they meet? J Nurs Adm 6:35, 1976

Index

Page numbers followed by f represent figures; page numbers followed by t represent tables.